Healing Through
Reiki

(An experience with Life Energy)

Bangalore
July 24, 2012

Healing Through
Reiki

(An experience with Life Energy)

Er. M.K. Gupta

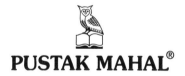

PUSTAK MAHAL®

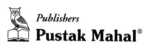

Publishers
Pustak Mahal®

J-3/16 , Daryaganj, New Delhi-110002
☎ 23276539, 23272783, 23272784 • *Fax:* 011-23260518
E-mail: info@pustakmahal.com • *Website:* www.pustakmahal.com

Sales Centre
• 10-B, Netaji Subhash Marg, Daryaganj, New Delhi-110002
  ☎ 23268292, 23268293, 23279900 • *Fax:* 011-23280567
  E-mail: rapidexdelhi@indiatimes.com
• **Hind Pustak Bhawan**
  6686, Khari Baoli, Delhi-110006
  ☎ 23944314, 23911979

Branches
Bengaluru: ☎ 080-22234025 • *Telefax:* 080-22240209
E-mail: pustak@airtelmail.in • pustak@sancharnet.in
Mumbai: ☎ 022-22010941, 022-22053387
E-mail: rapidex@bom5.vsnl.net.in
Patna: ☎ 0612-3294193 • *Telefax:* 0612-2302719
E-mail: rapidexptn@rediffmail.com
Hyderabad: *Telefax:* 040-24737290
E-mail: pustakmahalhyd@yahoo.co.in

© **Author**

ISBN 978-81-223-0114-4

9th Edition: June 2011

Printed at : Param Offsetters, Okhla, New Delhi-110020

Contents

Preface

Most of the people believe that we have only one body i.e. this physical body which is visible to the eye. But the fact is that we have many invisible bodies also which interpenetrate the physical body and are constituted of much finer matter as compared to physical matter. One such body in the immediate neighbourhood of physical body is our vital body or energy body or pranic body. It provides energy to the physical body and is the basis of all movements and activities taking place wihtin our physical body. Any disturbance in the energy body affects our physical body.

The same energy or prana which moves through our body also moves in the outer cosmos as cosmic prana in a purer form. Reiki is the science of healing of energy body using this cosmic life energy. Reiki Healer works as a channel for this healing. The removal of energy imbalance by such healing in any portion of the energy body automatically leads to healing in the corresponding part of the physical body.

In order to facilitate more scientific understanding of Reiki healing by the readers, I have first explained briefly about the anatomy of energy body, chakras, nadis, Aura and energy imbalance in the body. I have constantly endeavoured to associate Reiki with our ancient great yoga science so that readers may not treat Reiki as something strange or magical (as most laymen tend to think), but understand it as an outcome of our great science of yoga presented now in a more scientific way.

May you enjoy and derive maximum benefit from the book.

–M.K. Gupta
Nuclear Science Centre
J.N.U. Campus, New Delhi-110067

Acknowledgement

I am greatly indebted to Master Choa Kok Sui and his pioneering work in the field of Pranic Healing.

I have found his book "Miracles through Pranic Healing" so inspiring that I had to rely extensively on the contents of the same in the preparation of the entire Chapter 11, and portions of other Chapters in this present work.

Though Reiki is different from Pranic Healing, the Pranic Healing principles and techniques are so unique, potent and profoundly simple, that if Reiki practitioners were to integrate Master Choa Kok Sui's Pranic Healing in their healing practices, they could produce faster and better healing results.

I acknowledge that the concepts, terms, and techniques of 'scanning', 'cleansing', 'energizing', 'stabilizing', and 'releasing or cutting', among others, which I have incorporated in my book, are the intellectual creation and property of Master Choa Kok Sui, and that his books are the premier, pioneering, and authoritative sources in the field of energy healing.

I also acknowledge that without Master Choa Kok Sui's work, I would not have been able to accomplish the writing of this book.

I therefore express my heartfelt gratitude and thanks to Master Choa Kok Sui for granting me the permission to borrow heavily from his work "Miracles through Pranic Healing" so that this present work can be completed.

−**M.K. Gupta**

1

Reiki — The Universal Life Energy

The word Reiki comes from two Japanese words–'Rei' meaning universal, and 'Ki' meaning life energy or life force. So Reiki is Universal Life Energy (or force). The whole universe or cosmos is filled with this invisible life force, and this is the basis for sustaining life and health of all living beings. All living beings are constantly bathing in this infinite energy and ingesting it inside them.

This life force animates all living beings. As long as something is alive, it has life force circulating through it. When it dies, then life force departs. If our life force is depleted and not flowing freely, we will be feeling low in health and mood and will be more vulnerable to illness. When it is high and flowing freely, we are healthy and in high spirits. Although life force is basically for energizing physical body it has a great effect on mind also through a mechanism which will be explained later.

The Chinese identified this energy as 'Chi', Indians as 'Prana' or vital energy, and Japanese as 'Ki'. This energy is normally available to us from the following means or sources:

1. Air
2. Sunlight
3. Earth

9

4. Food
5. Water
6. Trees
7. Open sky (ether)

The more fresh and natural the above substances are, the better the quality and magnitude of Prana imparted by them. So, we can see that this energy has five aspects (or 'Panch Prana') corresponding to five elements of nature (Air, Water, Fire, Earth, Ether). When we are in physical contact with nature e.g. in the sun, enjoying natural bodies of water and lush vegetation, climbing on rock or feeling the wind embracing us, we are absorbing this vital life force energy. Such deep nourishment from nature relaxes and rejuvenates. Fresh natural foods and trees also give us a lot of prana and rejuvenate us because they constantly absorb the prana from these five elements of nature. You might have observed how relaxing and rejuvenating it is to lie under the shade of a big tree even in extreme summer.

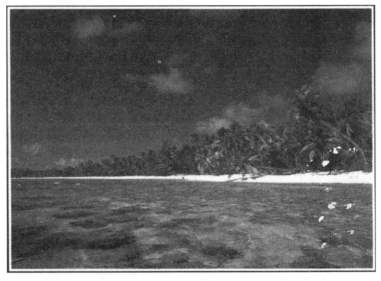

Fig. 1: 'Ki' or 'Prana' is Abundantly Available in Nature

The universal life energy enters inside us through our Crown Chakra. Although Reiki energy is naturally available to all living beings from birth, later due to various lifestyle defects, mental stresses and negative attitudes, its spontaneous flow is obstructed because of distortion of natural healing connection. However, through a confidential process of Reiki initiation or attunement by a Reiki initiating master, the blocked energy channels are reopened and Reiki energy again starts flowing freely. It is the initiation process that sets Reiki apart from other forms of pranic or energy healing.

Meditation is another way of dipping into this life force energy. But here the source of this life force energy is different and known as 'Kundalini' which will be explained further at the appropriate place in this book.

Although healing through life energy in some form or the other is as old as the advent of human

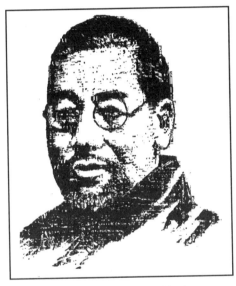

Fig. 2: Dr. Mikao Usui

civilization, Reiki in its present form was rediscovered by Dr. Mikao Usui of Japan about a hundred and seventy-five years ago.

11

2

Our Energy Body

Surrounding our physical body there is another body which interpenetrates it and extends beyond it by a few inches. This invisible luminous body which follows the contour of the physical body is called the 'Energy Body'. This is also known as Bioplasmic body or Pranic body or Vital body or Etheric body or Etheric double, and it is the exact duplicate of physical body. The projected part of this body beyond the physical body is also called 'Health Aura'.

This energy body is non physical in nature and is made of invisible etheric matter. Some people prefer to call it semi physical also as through specialized means, it can be seen with physical eyes and also captured on photographic film (e.g. Kirlian photography). Both the bioplasmic body (or the energy body) and the physical body are so closely related that what affects one, affects the other. By healing the energy body, the visible physical body gets healed automatically.

The function of energy body is to absorb, distribute and energize the physical body with 'prana' through a network of chakras or energy centres and 'nadis'. Chakras are very important parts of the energy body. Just as the physical body has major and minor organs, the energy body has major, minor and mini chakras. The prana collected by these chakras from the Ether, Air, Sun, Water or Earth is distributed through the bioplasmic channels in the physical body. These bioplasmic channels are also called 'Nadis' (Indian terminology) or 'meridians' (Chinese terminology). Pranic body has its own complex anatomy just like physical body and forms a separate body of knowledge in ancient yoga literature.

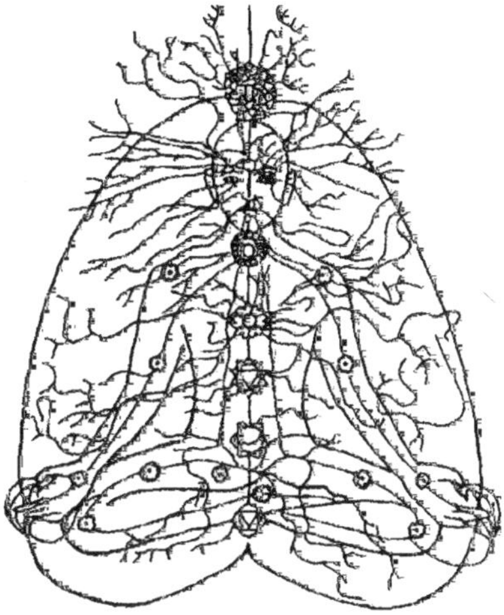

Fig. 2A: Ancient Concept of Pranic Body

Nadis in Yoga Science

Ancient yoga books speak of about 72,000 such 'nadis' or bioplasmic channels through which 'Ki' or 'prana' flows and is distributed all over the body. However out of these 72,000 nadis, three are supposed to be the major 'nadis' as mentioned below which feed the other nadis.

1. *'Ida' nadi (or lunar channel)* runs along the left side of spine. It starts from the lowest energy centre, and terminates in left nostril. Ida nadi is said to be cooling in nature.

2. *'Pingala' nadi (or solar channel)* runs along the right side of spine. It starts from the lowest energy centre and terminates in right nostril. Pingala nadi is said to be 'heating' in nature.

3. *'Sushumna' nadi (or the central Channel)* runs through the centre of spinal column. It starts from the lowest energy centre and goes right up to the top of the head (Crown Chakra).

Ida, Pingala and Sushumna may be considered as the main cables of nadi network like we have main and branch cables in electrical distribution network.

Chinese Meridians and Acupressure Points

In Chinese acupuncture or acupressure system, the pranic flow in these nadis is manipulated by applying pressure on some selective points in these nadis or meridians. Normally these acupuncture points are located where nadis or meridians come close to the surface of the body. Such pointed pressure redistributes the congested prana or excess prana in the diseased part to other parts of the body. In this way blocked meridians or bioplasmic channels are cleansed or opened and energy becomes free flowing leading to restoration of health.

Chinese speak of 26 main meridians alongwhich chi (or life energy) flows in the body. This calculation of meridians has something to do with the five elements. Five elements indicate five different modes in which this life energy manifests itself in the universe and inside our body. Each element governs a meridian or organ function in the body. Now the calculation of 26 meridians based on five elements is as follows.

Five elements have a pair of meridians each, one yin and one yang, except for fire which has two pairs. Hence from this consideration, no. of meridians $= 5 \times 2 + 2$ (extra for fire) $= 12$.

Now all twelve meridians are bilateral (i.e. on both sides of body from the centre line). Hence total meridians $= 12 \times 2 = 24$. Two extra meridians are usually included with the twelve organ meridians; the Governing vessels which is a kind of reservoir of 'yang' energy and controls all yang organ meridians and the conception vessel meridian which is its 'yin' counterpart. So this gives total of $24 + 2 = 26$ meridians.

Some distinctive feature of these acupuncture meridians are as follows–

1. One end of each meridian invariably lies either in hand or in foot.

2. Yin meridians normally run in front (or inside) of the body and energy travels upwards in them either towards the head or to fingers of the hands.

Yang meridians normally run at the back (or outside) of the body and energy travels downwards in them.

3. The intensity of flow of life energy in a particular meridian is not the same throughout the day. It increases and decreases in a cyclic fashion so that the energy passes from one meridian to the other in a sequence giving rise to most active time of a meridian (see table of meridians on page no. 19).

4. The paired meridians (Yin and Yang) run close to each other and their functions are complementary.

5. Acupuncture points are places on the meridians where the 'Chi' or 'Ki' can be most easily accessed and manipulated in the meridian.

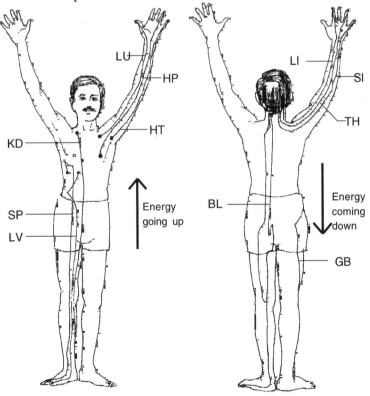

Fig. 2B: 'Yin' Meridians   *Fig. 2C: 'Yang' Meridians*

6. All acupuncture points on a meridian are connected. When you press sn acupuncture point on a meridian, you are influencing the flow of ki throughout the meridian.

7. Points near the ends of a meridian are often the most powerful in removing blocks or relieving pain along the course of that meridian.

See table of meridians at the end of chapter which gives the salient features of all the meridians.

Health Aura

From the surface of the physical body bioplasmic rays are projecting perpendicularly. These rays are called health rays, and sum of these health rays is called 'Health Aura'. The health aura follows the contour of the physical body and functions as a protective shield for the body from the germs and diseased bioplasmic matter in the surrounding area. The germs can be seen as being repelled and carried away by the outrush of pranic force. If a person is weakened, the health rays droop. Then the whole body becomes susceptible to infection and the capacity of health rays to repel toxins, germs, diseased pranic energy is greatly diminished. When the body gets diseased, there can be seen corresponding pranic leaks, holes, hollows or dark/black spots in the health aura of the person.

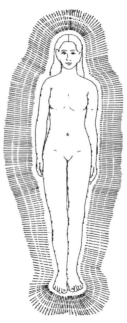

Fig. 3:
The Health Aura and its Health Rays

(Courtesy: "Miracles through Pranic Healing" by Master Choa Kok Sui for this fig. and the adjoining text matter).

16

Energy Body — A Link Between Mind and Physical Body:

Energy body is the link between mind and physical body and is greatly affected by various physical and mental factors taking place in our being. So, we can say that prana (or energy), mind and body act and react on one another.

At any moment in one's body, not only is matter being pushed about through veins and arteries or airways and changing its state according to varying bodily needs but energy (Prana or Ki) changes are also taking place accordingly. Energy is being consumed in one place and produced or stored up in another. It is being shifted from this point to that point resulting in a net movement of energy. Similarly the activities of the various chakras also keep on varying depending on bodily demands. For example, when we are in a danger and want to run away, the following chakras become overactive and coordinate with each other effectively.

1. *Swadhisthana chakra and kidney chakra* (minor chakra under Swadhisthana chakra) become active and cause adrenal glands to secrete more adrenaline.

2. *Ajna chakra* (or third eye chakra) becomes active and it activates the brain for necessary responses and generating necessary biochemicals and neurotransmitters. Since Ajna chakra is the master chakra, it has to be active in any case to organize the response of all other chakras.

3. *Solar plexus chakra* gets activated and in turn activates **liver chakra** (minor chakra under solar plexus chakra) to release more of sugar into blood stream for extra energy.

4. *Solar plexus chakra* and *Hara chakra* may also initiate bowel and bladder movements to get rid of waste matter instantly.

17

5. Messages from the *Spleen chakra* (minor chakra under solar chakra), *Hara or Swadhisthana chakra and Root or Muladhara chakra* contract blood vessels in the stomach and on the periphery of the body (skin) to reduce blood flow in these areas so that in case of injury, blood loss is minimized.

So you can see the complex and coordinated action of various chakras and nadis to meet a certain demand of the body. In fact, pranic body has an extremely complex anatomy and physiology and forms a distinct body of knowledge in yoga science.

Table of Meridian

S.N.	Name of Meridian	Yang/Yin	Element	Starts at	Ends at	Route of Meridian	Most active time	Physical organs/ system controlled	Negative Emotion	Positive Emotion
1.	Lung (LU)	Yin	Metal	Front of Shoulder	Thumb in hand	Front of arm	3-5 A.M.	Lungs, respiration skin	Sadness, Grief depression	Letting go
2.	Large Intestine (LI)	Yang	Metal	Tip of Index Finger	Nose tip	Outside of arm, top of shoulder	5-7 A.M.	Elimination of solid waste Cleansing, Detoxifying	"	"
3.	Stomach (ST)	Yang	Earth	Face (just below eyes)	2nd toe on top of foot	Face, Chest, front of thigh, shin bone	7-9 A.M.	Digestion of food	Worry and self pity	Openness and fairness to self & others
4.	Spleen (SP)	Yin	Earth	Side of big toe in foot	Side of chest (near arm pit)	Inner legs, Groin Ribs	9-11 A.M.	Spleen functions (storing blood, forming antibodies & W.B.C.) Pacreas functioning (Digestion blood sugar control), Menstruation	"	"
5.	Heart (HT)	Yin	Fire	Arm pit	Little finger in hand	Front of arm (towards inner side)	11A.M.-1P.M.	Heart & Circulation	Impatience, hatred, cruelty, arrogance hastiness, violence, bigotry	Joy, love, learning respect, honesty sincerity, radiance
6.	Small Intestine (SI)	Yang	Fire	Little finger	Face (front of ear)	Back of arm, Back of shoulders	1-3 P.M.	Assimilation of food, shoulder blades and joints	"	"
7.	Bladder (BL)	Yang	Water	Inner corner of eye socket	Little toe in each foot	Back of neck, upper & lower back, back of buttocks & legs	3-5 P.M.	Neck, Back, Buttocks, back of thighs, calves, bladder functioning. It has points which control all internal organs	Fear	Gentleness and wisdom

Contd.

19

S.N.	Name of Meridian	Yang/Yin	Element	Starts at	Ends at	Route of Meridian	Most active time	Physical organs/system controlled	Negative Emotion	Positive Emotion
8.	Kidney (KD)	Yin	Water	Sole (foot)	Front of chest	Side of foot, Inner leg, chest	5-7 P.M.	Sexual vitality stamina, Bones, Ears	Fear	Gentleness and Wisdom
9.	Heart Protector (HP) or Pericardium	Yin	Fire	Pectoral muscle in chest	Middle finger in hand	Front of arm	7-9 P.M.	Heart protection, circulation, sexual function		
10.	Triple Heater (TH)	Yang	Fire	Ring finger (4th finger) in hand	Temporal region in head	Along arm, shoulder sides of neck, around ear	9-11 P.M.	Respiration (upper warmer) Digestion (middle warmer) Elimination (Lower warmer)		
11.	Gall Bladder (GB)	Yang	Wood	Hollow at outside of eye socket	4th toe in foot	Top of shoulder, side of trunk, side of buttock and leg	11 P.M.- 1 A.M.	Gall bladder, flexibility & strength of tendons and ligaments, eyes, neck and shoulders	Anger	Kindness Decision making, will power
12.	Liver (LV)	Yin	Wood	Big toe top in foot	Liver	Inside of leg, reproductive organ	1-3 A.M.	Eyes, Nervous system, digestion of fats, liver problems, nails, muscles, tendors, reproductive system	Anger	"
13.	Conception Vessel (CV)	Yin	—	Tip of tongue	Perineum	Front of the body in the centreline		These meridians govern all other organ meridians. They balance these meridians by normalizing their energy excess or deficiencies.		
14.	Governing Vessel (GV)	Yang	—	Perineum	Upper Palate in mouth	Back of body in the centreline. Runs up the spine and over the skull to the upper palate				

3

Chakras (or Energy Centres)

Chakra is a Sanskrit word which means circle, wheel, something round and spinning. As already mentioned, etheric body or energy body has several chakras or energy centres which absorb and distribute prana throughout the body through a network of minor and mini chakras and nadis. Major chakras may be considered like main power stations from where the main supply goes to other areas. Minor and mini chakras may be considered as sub-power stations supplying power to localized areas. For example, we have very important minor chakras at our palm and sole, and mini chakras on finger and toes. Some of the other minor chakras are at the location of elbow, knee, armpit, liver, kidney, spleen etc. Nadis may be considered equivalent to electrical cables and wires through which prana flows.

There are many chakras in the body but the major chakras (seven in number) form an energy circuit along the axis of the spine in the region of five major nervous plexus. These chakras act as intermediaries receiving energy from higher levels and transmitting it throughout the body. At the location of major chakras, three major nadis Ida, Pingala and Sushumna meet together forming these centres of concentrated pranic energy.

There is another important function of these chakras which is less understood, that is, these energy centres act as an intermediary or bridge between the physical body and astral body transmitting the impressions between these two vehicles. In other words, these are points of connection between these two vehicles of man. Once we understand this, we can easily realize how mind and body affect each other. What happens is that any mental reaction or impulse or emotion first creates vibrations in the astral body. These vibrations are then transmitted through the etheric or energy body to the physical body. This is how mental states affect the physical body. In the similar fashion any disturbance in the physical body gets transmitted to the astral body through etheric body thus affecting the mind.

These chakras or wheels are perpetually rotating. However, in the undeveloped person, they are usually in comparatively sluggish motion. In a more evolved man, they may be glowing and pulsating with living light resembling miniature suns, so that an enormously greater amount of energy passes through them. In a newborn baby they are tiny little circles like a one paisa coin, little hard discs scarcely moving at all and only faintly glowing.

The chakras vary in size from about two inches in dia (in undeveloped person) to about six inches dia (in developed persons). They project about quarter of an inch outside the skin of the body. To a clairvoyant sight they appear as vortices or saucer like depressions on the surface of etheric body. Minor and mini chakras are lesser in diameter than major chakras (minor chakras—one to two inch dia, mini chakras—less than one inch dia). Hence it may be understood that the chakras are not simply inside the body. They interpenetrate and extend beyond the physical body. Nadis radiate out of chakras like spokes of a wheel.

Major chakras are seven in number. They correspond to some major endocrine glands and nerve plexus in the physical body to which they are proximate. It may be noted that these physical counterparts of chakras play a major role in influencing the health of human body, and they easily affect the chakras and are also easily affected by the malfunctioning of the corresponding chakra.

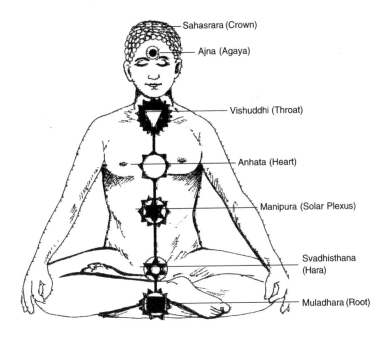

Fig. 4: Seven Major Chakras

The characteristics of these seven major chakras are presented in the tabular form in the next pages.

Description of Seven Major Chakras

Sl. No.	Name of Chakra	Location	Element	Colour	Corresponding Nerve plexus	Corresponding Endocrine Gland	Physical organs controlled	Mental aspects governed	Diseases due to malfunctioning of Chakra	Remarks
1.	Mooladhara Chakra (or Root or Base Chakra)	Base of the Spine	Earth	Red	Root plexus or Pelvic plexus or Coccygeal plexus	Adrenal	1. Muscular & Skeletal system 2. Spine 3. Adrenal glands 4. The production & quality of blood 5. Body heat 6. General vitality 7. Growth of children 8. Kidneys	Self protection, survival instinct, fear, insecurity	1. Arthritis 2. Spinal ailments 3. Blood ailments 4. Cancer (Bone cancer, Leukemia) 5. Allergy 6. Growth problem 7. Low vitality 8. Slow healing of wounds & broken bones	Persons with healthy root Chakra tend to be robust and healthy, full of vitality. Persons with weak Root Chakra tend to be weak and drained of vitality. Old people usually have depleted Root Chakra
2.	Swadhisthana Chakra (or Hara or Sacral or Sexual Chakra)	Near Sacrum or Pubic Area and slightly below navel	Water	Red—Orange	Sacral plexus or Hypogastric plexus or Aortic plexus	Gonads	1. Sex glands (ovaries, testicles) 2. Sexual organs (incl Prostate glands, Seminal Vesicles, Cowper glands) 3. Kidneys 4. Adrenal glands 5. Controls B.P. 6. Large intestines (colon) 7. Bladder, Rectum (excretion) 8. Uterus	Desire & craving for sexual & other sensual pleasures, seat of negative feeling of guilt, hurt & frustration	1. Sex related problems 2. High B.P 3. Back problems 4. Kidney problems 5. Bladder ailments 6. Constipation	It transmits vital energy throughout body via spleen chakra and back Hara chakra

Sl. No	Name of Chakra	Location	Element	Colour	Corresponding Nerve plexus	Corresponding Endocrine Gland	Physical organs controlled	Mental aspects governed	Diseases due to malfunctioning of Chakra	Remarks
3.	Manipura Chakra (or Solar Plexus Chakra)	Slightly above Navel & below ribs	Fire	Yellow	Solar Plexus or Coeliac Plexus	Pancreas	1. Stomach 2. Intestines 3. Spleen 4. Gall bladder 5. Diaphragm 6. To some degree adrenal glands, heart, lungs 7. Liver 8. Pancreas	Ego; Craving for name, fame, status, power, control; high ambitions and aggressive-ness; negative emotions like anger, jealousy, envy, hatred, greed, violence, cruelty	1. Digestive disorders 2. Ulcer 3. Constipation 4. Diabetes 5. Hepatitis 6. Jaundice 7. Colitis & Diorrhoea 8. Skin problem & allergies, 9. Heart problems & high B.P 10. Asthma	
4.	Anahata Chakra (or Heart Chakra)	Centre of chest at the height of heart	Air	Green	Cardiac Plexus	Thymus	1. Heart 2. Lungs 3. Thymus gland 4. Circulatory system	Love and compassion, centre of higher & refined emotions	1. Heart & circulatory ailments 2. Lung ailments (Bronchitis, asthma, tubercu-losis etc)	This Chakra is the end receiving point of Reiki energy from where it is distributed to arms and hands
5.	Vishuddhi Chakra (or Throat Chakra)	Hollow of Throat	Ether (Space or Akasa)	Blue	Pharyngeal Plexus or Cervical Plexus or Brachial Plexus	Thyroid	1. Throat, 2. Voice box (Larynx), 3. Airtube (Trachea), 4. Thyroid & Para-thyroid glands, 5. Lymphatic system, 6. Arms, hands, 7. Mouth tongue, 8. Neck	Communication, speech, selfexpre-ssion, creativity (musical & artistic talents etc), Aesthetics	Throat related diseases like. 1. Goitre 2. Sore throat 3. Speech or voice problems 4. Tonsilitis 5. Cervical pain	Strength of a person in his speech comes from Vishuddhi Chakra. Shouting, anger and use of foul language full of ego blocks this Chakra

25

Contd...

Sl. No	Name of Chakra	Location	Element	Colour	Corresponding Nerve plexus	Corresponding Endocrine Gland	Physical organs controlled	Mental aspects governed	Diseases due to malfunctioning of Chakra	Remarks
6	Ajna Chakra (or Brow or Third Eye Chakra)	Between the eyebrows	—	Indigo	Cavernous Plexus or Nasociliary Plexus	Pituitary	1. Hypothalmus 2. Pituitary & other endocrine glands 3. Autonomic Nervous System & Lower brain 4. Left eye 5. Ears 6. Nose	Intuition, Intellect, Occult powers/ E.S.P (e.g. Clairvoyance, telepathy etc.)	1. Diseases related to endocrine glands 2. Diseases related to Autonomic Nervous System (A.N.S) & lower brain 3. Diseases related to sight, hearing & smell 4. Sinusitis, swollen adenoids	It is called the master chakra and controls all other major chakras
7.	Sahasrara Chakra (or Crown Chakra)	Top of Head	—	Violet White	—	Pineal	1. Pineal gland 2. Upper or higher Brain 3. Right eye	Cosmic consciousness, self-realization	Diseases related to pineal gland and the cerebral cortex	It is also the entry point for Reiki energy. Sahasrara chakra is seen in meditation as a one thousand petalled lotus. Upon enlightenment, it looks like a burning bundle of flames

26

Note: Some of material in this table has been taken from Master Choa Kok Sui's famous book 'Miracles through Pranic Healing'. We convey our gratitude to them.

Some Useful Notes about Chakras

1. Colour mentioned against each chakra is the most predominant colour because a mixture of colours can be observed sometimes. Moreover these are not physical colours which you can see with physical eyes but these are astral colours and most closer counterparts of physical colours and are seen while chakras are perceived with trance vision.

2. Every chakra (except root and crown chakra) has two portions: (a) Front, (b) Back. These portions serve their corresponding parts. While front portion chakra is accessed from the front of the body, back portion of chakra is accessed from back of the body. (See Fig. 5). Then each chakra has left and right side.

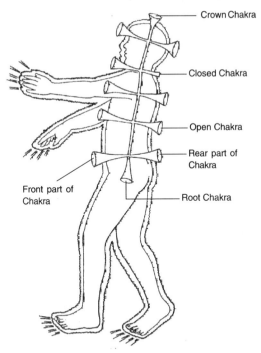

*Fig. 5: Front and Rear,
Open and Closed Chakras*

3. Every physical and mental activity influences the sensitivity and performance of the chakras. When chakras become blocked or insensitive due to catches (adverse physical and mental factors), central channel (Sushumna nadi) remains closed and Kundalini can't ascend through it.

4. Chakras, in fact the whole bioplasmic body, are greatly influenced by the mental activity especially the negative emotions in the mind. Anger and intense worry devitalize the whole bioplasmic body so that the body becomes susceptible to all kinds of diseases. This is the reason why a person feels so exhausted after an intense anger or altercation. An emotional trauma may damage a chakra in the same way as a serious physical disease.

5. Chakras rotate clockwise and the speed of rotation of lower level chakras is less and that of higher level chakras is high. The rate of vibration in each chakra in turn affects the functioning of glands and organs to which it connects, thus influencing the entire body. When chakras malfunction, their speed or frequency of rotation gets disturbed from their optimum value.

6. The solar plexus chakra has strong influence on the physical heart and the front heart chakra. Malfunctioning of the solar plexus chakra may cause the front heart chakra and the physical heart to malfunction. The front heart chakra is closely connected to the front solar plexus chakra by several big bioplasmic channels and is also energized by the front solar plexus chakra to a certain degree. Patients with heart problems usually have malfunctioning solar plexus chakra. Like heart and solar plexus, the following chakras also show interrelation and form pairs:

Throat Chakra and Hara Chakra

Ajna Chakra and Root Chakra

It is observed that in paired chakras, when we give energy to one, the other chakra also gets energized. Hence it is advisable to treat the paired chakra also when you are treating any chakra for any ailment.

7. The solar plexus chakra is quite sensitive to emotion, tension and stress. For instance, anger, worry, prolonged irritation and frustrations may result in pranic depletion around the solar plexus chakra or may manifest as pranic congestion around the solar plexus chakra and front heart chakra. In the first case, it manifests itself as indigestion or loose bowel movement. In the long run, it may manifest itself as ulcer or gall bladder problem. In the second case, it may manifest as heart enlargement or many heart related problems. Solar plexus chakra is also affected by too much thinking about food and taking bad food like alcohol, too much greasy food, etc.

8. If a person's vital body is strong then his probability of contracting a disease due to external factors like bacteria/virus, pollutants etc. is greatly reduced because body's aura and defence mechanism will easily counter the effects of external irritants.

9. Some chakras are sites or centres of psychic faculties. Activation of certain chakras may result in the development of these psychic faculties or siddhis. For example, activation of Ajna chakra results in powers of clairvoyance, clairaudience, etc. Activation of Palm chakra (minor chakra) results in sensing subtle pranic energy.

Note: Courtesy 'Miracles through Pranic Healing' by Master Choa Kok Sui for matter explained in point no. 6 & 7 on page no. 28 & 29.

10. Too much planning, too much thinking, too much sensuality and taking too much drugs, alcohol exhaust the 'Swadhisthana' or Hara chakra.

11. Inhalation of smoke particularly cigarette smoke and use of foul language and shouting damages Vishuddhi Chakra or Throat centre. The best way to clear this chakra is to become humble and talk sweetly to people giving due respect.

12. If one has wobbling eyes then the Ajna chakra gets blocked. If one's Ajna chakra is alright then the eyes remain alright. They emit love wherever they glance. This chakra also gets cleared by developing the quality of forgiveness. People who are unable to forgive their enemies catch on this Ajna chakra. When Ajna chakra opens, Kundalini can pass through it to Sahasrara chakra.

13. A strong back Ajna is essential for good sleep whereas overactive Ajna hinders sleep.

14. Yogis who perceived these chakras in deep meditation saw that they resembled lotus flowers of different shades with different number of petals. Each chakra has a certain number of petals which correspond to sub-plexus just as main chakra corresponds to major plexus. For example, Swadhisthana chakra having six petals corresponds to Aortic plexus as major nerve plexus and six sub-plexus corresponding to six petals. Figure 6 gives the number of petals in each chakra.

15. Lower three chakras (Root, Hara and Solar plexus) indicate lower level of consciousness in the scale of evolution while higher chakras (Heart, Throat, Ajna, Sahasrar) correspond to higher levels of consciousness. When a person's energy is primarily focussed on the lower level chakras, his mental

Sahasrara Chakra
The thousand-petalled crown chakra corresponds to the Absolute. When Kundalini reaches this point, the yogi attains samadhi or superconsciousness.

Ajna Chakra
This chakra has two petals. Seat of the mind, its mantra is OM.

Vishuddhi Chakra
This chakra has sixteen petals. Its element is ether and its mantra, Ham.

Anahata Chakra
This Chakra has twelve petals. Its element is ether and its mantra, Yam.

Manipura Chakra
This chakra has ten petals. Its element is fire and its mantra, Ram.

Swadhishthana Chakra
This chakra has six petals. Its element is water and its mantra, Vam.

Muladhara Chakra
This chakra has four petals. Its element is earth and its mantra, Lam.

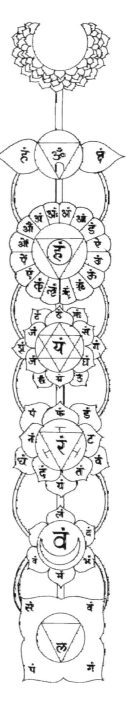

Fig. 6: Mantra, Yantra and Number of Petals for Each Chakra

31

attitudes or traits are governed by the psychological aspects of these chakras as mentioned in the table of chakras. Similarly when a person operates from the level of higher chakras, his mental traits correspond to the psychological aspects of these chakras as mentioned in the table. This happens only when the energy is allowed to leave the domain of the lower level chakras and enter in the domain of higher level chakras.

16. Each chakra is associated with a mantra and yantra (geometrical figure). If we focus on these mantras and yantras, we can awaken that chakra easily (See Fig. 6).

Representation of Chakras at Various Points in the Body

The seven main chakras are also represented in our hands, feet and head as shown in the following figure. Hence by feeling the sensations in these parts of the body, we can check the condition of a chakra. For example, an obstruction in the right heart chakra will show itself as heat, tingling, numbness or pulsation in the little finger of the right hand. When chakras are cleared, we feel cool vibrations like a soothing breeze coming from these fingers or from other parts to which these chakras correspond. There is, however slight variations in the representation of these chakras among various schools of psychic healing.

Conversely, by giving vibrations or energy to these representative areas of chakras, main chakras also get cleared and energized.

Problems in chakras can also show themselves in other parts of the body. For instance, our solar plexus chakra is also expressed in our knees and elbows. By giving vibrations to these representative areas of chakras, chakras are also cleared. Similarly, our Mooladhara chakra is also represented on nose tip. Ancient yogic texts state that by doing 'Trataka' on nose tip, one can awaken his Mooladhara Chakra.

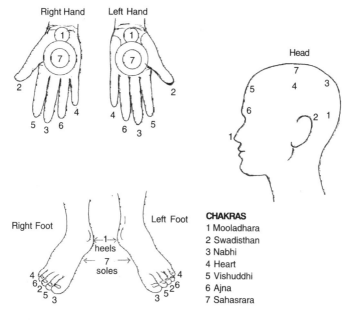

Fig. 7: Representation of Chakras at Various Points

CHAKRAS
1 Mooladhara
2 Swadisthan
3 Nabhi
4 Heart
5 Vishuddhi
6 Ajna
7 Sahasrara

33

4

Energy Imbalance—Root Cause of All Problems

Disease of any kind whether physical, mental or psychosomatic indicates some imbalance inside us. This imbalance is nothing but imbalance in the energy body. It is interesting to note that this life energy or prana is linked both to body and mind. It is an intermediary or bridge between the two and this only explains how physical body affects the non-physical mind and how non-physical mind affects the body.

Anything happening in the body affects the mind through the agency of prana. Similarly, anything happening in the mind also affects the body through the agency of prana. When body and mind are functioning in a healthy manner, energy or prana is flowing freely and uniformly everywhere. There is no blockage, congestion or depletion of prana anywhere. Hence there is no disease.

However, when body and mind are being misused, functioning unhealthily, abnormally or are overexerted, energy flow becomes imbalanced, i.e. energy becomes blocked and congested at one place, depleted at another place leading to some kind of disease (dis-ease) in body.

Physical Factors Causing Imbalance

Now at the bodily level there are many factors by which we disturb the natural and healthy flow of prana. Some of them are listed below:

1. Irregular lifestyle (e.g. sleeping, waking, eating at irregular and odd timings)

2. Overeating, oversleeping

3. Use of alcohol, smoking (tobacco), tea, coffee, narcotic drugs

4. Faulty diet (Rajasik & Tamsik foods)

5. Overexertion

6. Overindulgence in sensual pleasures

7. Excessive talking/gossiping/roaming un-necessarily here and there

8. Faulty postures, faulty breathing

9. Living in polluted, noisy environment. Living in extremely hot/cold/humid environment

10. Excessive company and mingling with people

11. Drugs and medication

In short, if any Rajasik or Tamsik activity disturbs the energy flow of the body then it generates negative energy. On the otherhand, Satwik lifestyle and activities promote the balanced and free flow of prana and generate positive energy. Whatever organs or systems get damaged due to the negative physical factors mentioned above, pranic flow in the corresponding nadis and chakras get disturbed.

Mental Factors Causing Imbalance

As mentioned earlier, just like physical factors, mental factors can also affect energy flow and damage chakras. If we want to sum up all the negative mental factors in two words, which disturb the flow of prana and health of chakras, those two words will be 'Negative thinking'. Now the next question comes 'why negative thinking arises'? The simple answer is-not accepting and understanding the things as they really are. The more the gap between the reality of things and your imagination/assumption about them, the more tense, nervous and anxious you will be.

Because of this huge gap between how things really are and what we imagine them to be, we are continually suppressing, rejecting and fighting with ourselves and outside world. This doesn't allow us to be integrated, whole and complete in our personality. We become a fragmented personality where one portion is going this way, another portion is going that way. The result is tension and conflict which doesn't allow energy to flow freely. As per yoga psychology, in such a state our unconsciousness is relatively vast and consciousness not well developed.

So, the first thing to do is to stop suppressing things and start seeing and understanding things from a broader perspective. We should start accepting and integrating everything into our consciousness avoiding nothing. This integration finally leads us to a state of unity, wholeness and completeness. Suppression brings about separation which creates loneliness, discomfort and a feeling of dis-ease. Whatever is suppressed and not integrated into our personality becomes alien to us and a constant source of disturbance. But as we develop, a process of integration takes place among all alienated or conflicting aspects of ourselves leading to increased happiness and satisfaction.

When our consciousness is fully developed, we finally reach that state of enlightenment and equilibrium from which all can be understood, appreciated and accepted. It is also to be noted that when consciousness is not fully developed and integrated, there is lot of egocentric move and selfishness in one's personality and lack of concern for others. But as consciousness gradually becomes expanded and integrated, we become less self-centered with more concern for others. This, in spiritual parlance, is also stated as moving from a state of separation (selfishness) to the state of unity (selflessness).

Now when the personality is not integrated, it is reflected in our behaviour in various forms as mentioned below:

(a) Negative emotions (e.g. anger, irritation, impatience, intolerance, fear, anxiety, worry, nervousness, hatred, jealousy, revengeful nature, hurry, over-ambition, restlessness, depression, sadness, hopelessness and helplessness, lack of confidence, etc.

(b) Desires and expectations.

(c) Craving and passion for name, fame, power, status, control, domination.

(d) Various 'Vikaras' like greed, attachment, selfishness, ego, etc.

(e) Unsteadiness and distractions in mind, inability to focus.

Now the most important question is how these negative mental factors affect our energy body and thence the physical body.

The explanation of this question is that these negative mental factors create corresponding vibrations in our astral body. Since astral body is connected to etheric body (or pranic body) at the point of chakras or energy centres, hence corresponding chakras get affected and start malfunctioning. Now the organs to which these chakras feed energy, also start malfunctioning as a result.

Mental feeling	Energy centre which is affected
1. Inability to love all universally	Heart chakra will be blocked
2. Lack of self-expression, inability to communicate and speak effectively	Throat chakra will be blocked
3. Excessive sex and sensory pleasures	Hara chakra will be blocked
4. Craving for name, fame, ego, power; domination and control over others; aggressiveness, anger, jealousy, hatred, impatience; violence, cruelty, harshness, exploitation	Solar Plexus chakra will be blocked
5. Compassion, love, kindness, sympathy for all, unity with creation	Heart chakra will be opened
6. Fear, insecurity, feeling threat to survival	Root chakra will be blocked and digestive disorders, knees, calves and feet will be affected (Refer Reiki positions)
7. Deep-rooted feelings of hurt and guilt	Hara and throat chakras as will be affected
8. Foul speech, shouting, showing disrespect to others	Throat chakra will be blocked
9. Humbleness and sweetness in talking with love and respect	Throat chakra will be opened
10. Unsteadiness of mind and eyes	Ajna chakra will be blocked

Mental feeling	Energy centre which is affected
11. Inability to forgive enemies	Ajna chakra will be blocked
12. Extreme helplessness and hopelessness	Paralysis, numbness of arms, hands and legs, Asthma
13. Over sensitiveness, suppression, restricted communication between you and world	Allergy, skin problems (Eczema, Acne, etc.)
14. Steadiness/concentration of mind and eyes	Ajna chakra will be opened
15. Forgiveness	Ajna chakra will be opened
16. Greediness, attachment	Hara chakra will be affected leading to constipation
17. Disharmony and non-adjustment in relationships with partner and other close relatives resulting in disappointment, frustration	Kidneys will be affected
18. Pent-up aggression, bitterness, hard feelings	Gallstones, kidney stone will be formed
19. Overthinking and over-planning	Swadhisthan (or Hara) chakra will be damaged
20. Fearlessness	Mooladhara chakara will be opened

The above table shows the relationship between the energy centres (or body part having this energy centre) and corresponding mental factors which influence them.

39

Energy Imbalance from Yogic Perspective

In yoga, the energy balance is explained in terms of activity of Ida, Pingala and Sushumna nadis, and it is very interesting to know about it. (Please refer Fig. 8 in this connection.)

Imbalance towards Left Side

As has been explained earlier, Ida nadi (or moon's channel) travels along the left side of the spine starting from the Muladhara chakra and ascending upto Ajna chakra. The

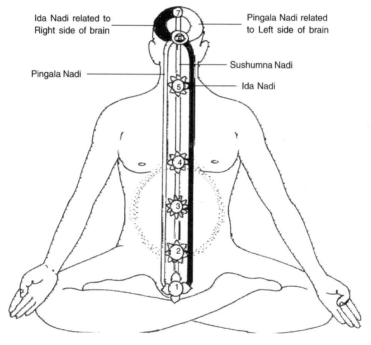

Ida Nadi related to Right side of brain

Pingala Nadi related to Left side of brain

Pingala Nadi

Sushumna Nadi

Ida Nadi

Fig. 8: Three Major Nadis

qualities assigned to this nadi are Tamoguna, past events and subconscious. It always brings to consciousness the memories of the past. The persons who are left sided (i.e. in whom Ida nadi mostly remains active) are those people who keep on thinking of the past, are very emotional, prefer darkness, avoid meeting people and are introverts. Such persons get various types of diseases of the left side. They become very lethargic, retreating into passivity and self-obsession which finally culminates in lunacy, epilepsy, senile decay.

Persons who are left sided should balance it with the right side by activity, work and action, discarding all ideas of self destruction and self pity. Our left side is represented on the whole left hand.

Imbalance towards Right Side

As has been mentioned, Pingala nadi or the sun channel runs along the right side of spine starting from Muladhara up to Ajna chakra. This nadi has qualities of Rajo Guna. It represents our desire for action (kriya shakti). It makes us think, work, plan and organize for the future events.

The symptoms of right sided persons are that they are very aggressive, over ambitious and dominating type. Right sided persons become very dry and lose all soft feelings. They are concerned only for their selfish material achievement and power over others. Blinded by ego, they take pride in exploiting and fooling the world. Such people get diseases of right side. Problems on Pingala nadi result largely from our presumption that it is we who are doing something while in fact all work is done only by Almighty God.

Any extreme physical or mental activity can paralyze our left emotional side and move us on to the right side so that we move into supraconscious (future) where we see visions like those induced by hallucinogenic drugs.

Overactive right side is brought into balance by moving the energy towards the centre, to Satoguna. Our right side is represented on our whole right hand.

Balance at the Centre

When the powers of both left (Ida nadi and Tamoguna) and right side (Pingla nadi and Rajoguna) are brought to balance, we get established in the centre or Satoguna.

The central channel or Sushumna nadi begins at Mooladhara and goes straight up to the highest chakra namely 'Sahasrara'. The qualities of this nadi are Sato guna, present centredness and superconsciousness. It is represented in both the hands. It is through this channel that we become superconscious and integrated into one whole. When Sushumna nadi gets opened, Kundalini can ascend in this central channel and go right up to Sahasrara chakra leading to our enlightenment. Doing regular meditation in thoughtless awareness (pure perception) and leading virtuous life is vital to opening of Sushumna.

Sushumna nadi is also called the channel of the Eternal present, where the only time is now. **In this way, we transcend time and space by opening of Sushumna and Kundalini awakening.**

Achieving the Balance of Nadis

In 'Sahaj Yoga' some simple techniques are suggested to achieve the balancing of right and left sides of the body as mentioned below:

(1) If a person is right sided then the energy of Ida nadi is raised by making ascending movements of the right hand along the right side and brought to the left side of the person's spine. (Fig. 9)

(2) If a person is left sided, i.e. apathetic and depressed, then the energy of Pingala nadi is raised by making ascending movements of the right hand along left side of the body and brought to the right side of the person's spine. (Fig. 10)

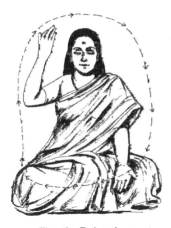

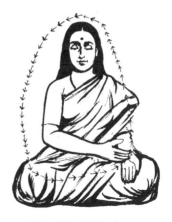

Fig. 9: Balancing
Overactive Right Side

Fig. 10: Balancing
Overactive Left Side

Clearing the Chakras

A chakra could also be cleared by simulating its clockwise rotation with the fingers of the right hand by a healer and asking the patient to keep his right hand on the afflicted chakra and keeping his left hand on the left knee with palms up and fingers open. In the science of prana, left hand is always used for receiving energy and right hand for imparting energy. Now depending on which side of chakra is afflicted— whether left side, right side, front or back, there can be slight variations accordingly in the healing.

There are other methods of clearing the chakras also, e.g. candling. It clears the chakras on the left side. Here a burning candle is moved up and down on the left side of spine. Similarly, there are other methods for clearing chakras like foot soaking in lukewarm salt water. Right side chakras are normally cleared by cold water treatment in the form of foot soaking in cold water. Foot soaking in river or sea water is said to clear Solar and Hara chakras. Sitting on mother earth or walking barefoot on the earth or grass clears Muladhara chakra. Putting hands on earth or in flowing river water or in lukewarm salt water is equally beneficial for clearing chakras. Salt has the special quality of breaking down the negative energy. Doing concentration or "Trataka" with open eyes on some object especially candle flame helps in awakening the Ajna chakra. *Even when in a normal way our mind is focussed and centered in some activity, it helps in activating Ajna chakra. Meditation is the strongest method for energizing Ajna chakra.*

Yoga science also speaks of reciting (mentally) specific mantras for awakening each chakra. This science is based on matching the subtle frequency of each chakra with subtle frequency of specific mantra so as to create resonance. However, since our subject is Reiki, we won't go into these details in this book.

Another technique of clearing chakra is by strengthening their qualities as mentioned in the table of chakras. As has been mentioned earlier, the chakras which are catching and blocked are only responsible for psychic and physical problems related to that chakra.

One of the easiest method to awaken chakras is to mentally focus your attention (with eyes closed) on them. To increase your concentration on a particular chakra you can imagine that you are breathing through that chakra (i.e. inhaling and exhaling through that chakra).

All the above information for clearing nadis and chakras is given here only for general enlightenment of the reader. However, since the purpose of this book is to cleanse the energy body through Reiki healing, the other chapters give the details of healing your energy body through Reiki. Nevertheless if you continue to use other techniques for balancing your energy body as described in this chapter and also in chapter titled 'Supporting aids for Reiki Practice', it will definitely do you more good.

5

Reiki Attunement

Reiki attunement is a process of empowerment that opens your crown, throat, heart and palm chakras and connects you to the unlimited source of Reiki energy. During the attunement, and for a time after, changes will be made by the attunement energy that open your system, enabling you to channel Reiki. These changes take place in the chakras, aura and also in the physical body. An emotional as well as toxic release can take place as part of this clearing process.

The Reiki initiation (or attunement) empowers us to be instruments to assist the healing process whenever we put our hands on ourselves or another. Performed by a traditionally trained Reiki master, the initiation enables us to access universal life energy easily and consistently. Initiation raises the student's energy field to a higher vibratory level activating fully the capacity to heal. Spending a brief time with each student, the Reiki master performs a sacred ceremony for each initiation based on the precise formula Dr. Usui (founder of the present form of Reiki Healing) discovered. This ritual finetunes, balances and aligns the student's energy body, empowering him to become a conduit for channelling universal life energy just like a radio being tuned to a specific frequency. The more spiritually advanced the master is, the higher the level of connection of the student with Reiki energy is. Universal life force is all around us. The initiation process tunes our energy fields so that we can receive this energy perfectly. The initiations sensitize the student's hands making them better able to conduct energy and detect energy flow. Such persons who have undergone process of Reiki attunenent are called Reiki channels and are fit for imparting healing to others and self.

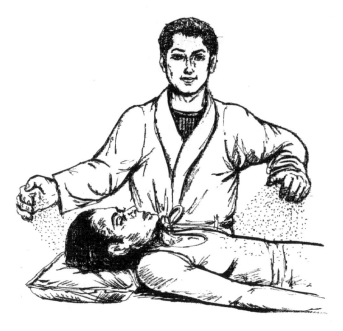

Fig. 11

As initiations raise the vibrations of our energy bodies, vitality increases and we are better able to protect our-selves against adverse environmental and situational circumstances. The flow of life force energy is contingent upon intention as well as bodily demand. However, the energy flows without constant focus or verbal repetition of intention. Intention to assist the healing process is implicit in the placing of our hands on our own body or another's. Nevertheless, there is no harm in consciously employing intention and awareness of the flow of life energy. Following the Reiki initiation, the universal life energy flows through our hands in response to our intention and the demand of the body's cells. The flow is nothing we can will or force because it depends on the cellular demand of the receiver's body. The healing happens as a result of the relationship between the receiver's energy field and the universal energy field mediated through the Reiki channel.

6

Basic Principles of Reiki Healing

1. Reiki can never do any harm.

One never need worry about whether to give Reiki or not. It is always helpful. It can never do harm.

2. Reiki also travels to other areas, apart from the place where hands are placed.

Reiki will not only treat the area where your hands are placed but will often travel to other areas of the body where it is needed. For example, when the hands are placed on the head, Reiki will treat the head but may also travel to the stomach. Similarly when you are treating the soles of the feet, Reiki can also flow above to your stomach and back.

3. Healer's energies are never depleted.

Reiki practitioner's energies are never depleted because it is not the healer's own energy which is going to the patient. It is the universal life energy which is going into the patient through the healer. Healer is simply acting as a conduit between universal life energy and the patient. In fact, giving the healing always increases one's energy instead of decreasing.

4. Reiki flow depends upon the demand of the body.

You can never give too little or too much Reiki. Reiki has its own instinctive intelligence which decides where to go and in what amount. The flow is nothing we can will or force because it depends on the cellular demand of the receiver's body. Therefore, all that is necessary for a Reiki channel or healer is simply to place his hands on the appropriate place and allow Reiki to work by remaining calm and relaxed.

5. Reiki treatment is equally effective for self and others.

In addition to treating others by Reiki, you can also treat yourself. It works just as well on yourself as on others. (Later in this book, hand positions for treating both your-self and others have been shown through suitable illustrations.)

6. Healing is not done by the healer. Healer is only a medium.

In the Reiki culture, it is strictly believed that you are your own healer. Healer is only creating a condition whereby your own healing can be accelerated. If you are diseased, it means that your own healing system is unbalanced right now and not properly open to receiving infinite life energy which is around us. Healer just does that by becoming a mediator. But it is to be kept in mind that finally it is you who are going to heal yourself and not anybody else.

7. No constant focus or verbal repetition is required for flow of Reiki.

Reiki energy flows without constant focus or any verbal repetition. After the Reiki initiation, simply putting the hands on the appropriate place with the intention of healing is enough to switch on Reiki flow. You can talk to someone or see TV while giving Reiki. However, if you consciously put your attention and awareness on the flow of Reiki, it is definitely better.

8. Feeling of warmth, coldness, pressure etc. during Reiki healing.

While giving Reiki, healers and patients feel different types of sensations which give important clues about the energy state of the patient's body. For example, while giving Reiki, healer feels hot and pressure in his hands. It means there is a resistance to flow of energy in patient's body because of blockage of energy channels. If the patient is feeling cold, it is because negative energy is going out from his body which makes him feel so. When the patient is feeling heaviness or pressure at some place while receiving Reiki, it means energy channels at that place are blocked because of which energy is not able move freely there and is applying pressure to push the blocked-up negative energy. However, after sometime the condition may normalize.

9. Reiki can also be given to animals and plants.

Animals and plants are survived by the same life energy which sustains us. Hence they (animals and plants) can also be given Reiki and treated.

10. Reiki is always given on asking.

Reiki is never forced on anyone. The patient should ask for healing from a Reiki Therapist. Resistance stops the free flow of Reiki. Further healee (or patient) shouldn't be kept in debt by doing free service. Rather healee should duly compensate for the time spent by therapist for healing.

11. Healer shouldn't be attached to the result.

Reiki therapist remains detached from the result of the healing. He only does the process to the best of his ability and with love and leaves the result in the hands of Divine, realizing that he is only a channel. Healing results depend on so many factors including 'Karmas' of the patient.

7

Preparing Hands for Energy Transfer in Reiki

There are three places in our body from where life energy flows outside abundantly. These are:

1. Hands   2. Feet   3. Eyes

In addition, we can also transmit life energy to someone by breathing upon him. In the case of transmission of life energy by eyes, one has to focus his eyes or visual attention on the area to be treated and energy goes there.

However, in Reiki we mostly make use of hands to impart energy to self and others as it is more convenient. The energy flow comes from above, down through the Crown Chakra, Third Eye Chakra, Throat Chakra, Heart Chakra and from there to the hands. There are two very important chakras located at the centre of each palm. Although they are considered minor chakras, they are very important. It is through the hand chakras that the prana is projected to the patient. Both the left hand and right hand chakras are capable of absorbing and projecting prana or Ki. Similarly there is a mini chakra in each finger. These chakras are also capable of absorbing and projecting prana.

Note: Courtesy 'Miracles through Pranic Healing' by Master Choa Kok Sui for matter explained in last para of this page.

After Reiki attunement, simply placing your hands on someone with the intention of giving Reiki will be enough to start it flowing. Reiki flows so easily that just thinking or talking about it turns it on. No great concentration or focus is required. You can go on talking to someone else or seeing TV while putting your hand on the affected part. However, it works better if you focus your awareness on the flow of Reiki, allowing your consciousness to merge with it. Be aware of the sensations in your hands such as warmth, tingling, vibrations, pulsations or a free flow of energy.

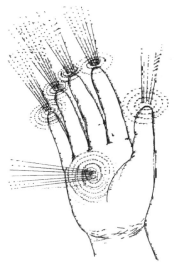

Fig. 12: Hand and Finger Chakras (energy centres)

(Courtesy: 'Miracles through Pranic Healing', by Master Choa Kok Sui for this fig. and some of the text matter on previous page 51.

A few simple tips however will prepare your hands better for giving Reiki. These are:

1. Wash and clean your hands properly before giving Reiki.

2. Relax your hands by opening and clenching your fists a few times and by jerking and shaking your hands a few times. Relaxation leads to freer energy flow in hands and more sensitiveness to subtle pranic energy.

3. Bring your awareness to the palm of your hand. This coupled with instructions given in S. No. 1 and 2 activates the hand chakra located at the centre of palms. By activating the hand chakras, one develops the ability to feel subtle energies. This is also called

sensitizing the hands. Once your hands are prepared, you can clearly sense the warmth of life energy flowing through them by bringing your hands near and far and by circling them facing each other as shown in the following figure. (Fig. 13)

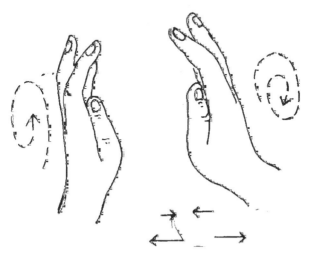

Fig. 13: Feeling Pranic Energy

4. When giving treatment, it is important to keep your fingers and thumb together. This will concentrate the energy and create a stronger flow. See Fig. 14.

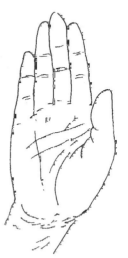

Fig. 14: Keeping Thumb and Fingers Together

Note: The term 'Sensitizing the hands' was originally coined by Master Choa Kok Sui and is, henceforth, being used widely by Pranic healers in their practice.

53

5. Hands should remain cupped for maximum energy flow (because of pyramid effect).

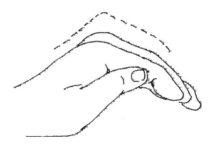

Fig. 15: Cupped Hand (Pyramid effect)

6. After Reiki treatment wash the hands properly with soap, alcohol, or salt water etc. Salt and alcohol have the property of disintegrating dirty bioplasmic matters etc. You can also jerk away and shake the hands in WC pan of toilet or in a vessel filled with salt water to throw away any negative energy which has stuck to your hand.

The most important way to increase the effectiveness of Reiki is to emanate it from love, compassion, kindness and with feeling of joy, cheerfulness and well being for others.

8

Full Body Reiki

Dr. Mikao Usui, founder of the present form of Reiki healing, discovered 31 points for full body Reiki healing treatment. These 31 points correspond to important major and minor chakras of the body and by giving Reiki treatment on these points, practically the whole body is covered for healing. In the body positions shown in the enclosed figures, 26 points are shown. As each leg has 5 points each, hence the total points become 31 if we count the 5 extra positions for another leg.

(A) Guidelines for Providing Reiki Treatment

The following points should be remembered while giving full body Reiki to self or other:

1. An average of three minutes of Reiki should be given on each point. But there will be no harm if this time is less or more. In some positions which are diseased you may have to give Reiki for more than 3 minutes for full healing.

2. The order of healing in full body Reiki should be followed as shown in the enclosed body positions from point 1 to 31. It is because this is the natural sequential flow of Reiki energy.

3. Reiki should never be given on top of head (Crown chakra) and on navel because these are the inlets or entry points of energy.

4. Thumb should not be apart from the fingers while giving Reiki. (See Fig. 14 in chapter 7)

5. Hands should be cupped for maximum energy flow. (See Fig. 15 in chapter 7)

6. If Reiki is given to others especially women, hands should be 2–3" away from the body while giving Reiki on Heart chakra.

7. Healer's and healee's legs/feet shouldn't be crossed. This interferes with free flow of energy.

8. Wash hands before giving healing.

9. Lying down position is preferable for giving Reiki to others. However, if any position requires it, change to a sitting or standing posture or face down lying position according to convenience of giving healing.

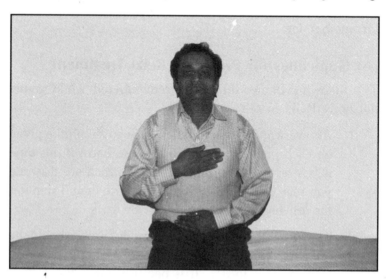

Fig. 16

10. At the end of Reiki treatments it is advisable to lie down with right hand on front Heart chakra and left hand on Front Hara. It is a very beneficial Reiki position in which left hand is symbolic of drawing negative energy from Hara while right hand is symbolic of providing energy to heart. If one sleeps in this position, he can have very soothing sleep. Similarly you can maintain this position while watching TV or simply sitting. So, you will be getting energy even while you are doing something else. Isn't it great! (See Fig. 16)

11. If in your own body, any part is difficult to touch or hold, you can beam Reiki to it as shown in Fig. 17. Closer the distance, the better it is. This will have the same effect as touch Reiki as explained in next point.

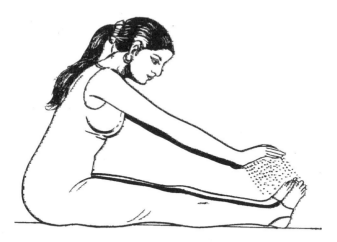

Fig. 17: Beaming of Reiki

12. It is not absolutely necessary to give Reiki by physical touch. You can also give Reiki with hands 1–4" away from the body with the standard hand positions. In this case, Reiki will first treat the aura and then enter

the physical body. Some people in fact prefer this because illness first exists in the aura before manifesting in the physical body. However, opinions vary among various people. Two examples are given below for illustration (Figs. 18 and 19).

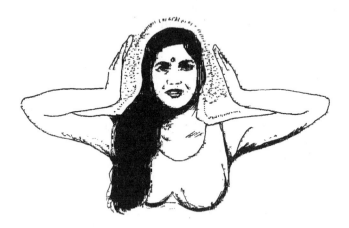

Fig. 18: Self Treatment without Touching

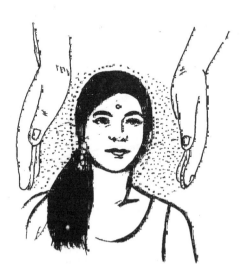

Fig. 19: Other's Treatment without Touching

13. While giving energy on Heart chakra, right hand should be below the left hand (i.e. right hand should touch the body) whereas at other positions there are no such restrictions, i.e. you can touch the body with either hand.

14. If possible, do 'sweeping' of energy body before giving regular Reiki treatment. It will help the body accept Reiki more fully. (See chapter 11 for details of 'Sweeping'.)

15. For giving Reiki to a small child, he can be taken in the lap. See Fig. 20, 21.

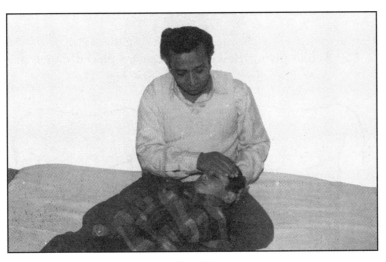

Fig. 20

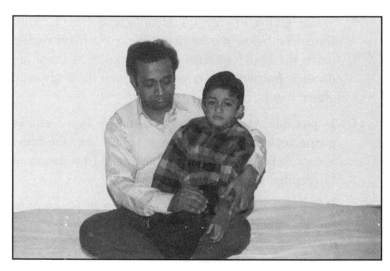

Fig. 21

16. While giving Reiki hands can be placed either one over the other or separate. See Fig. 22.

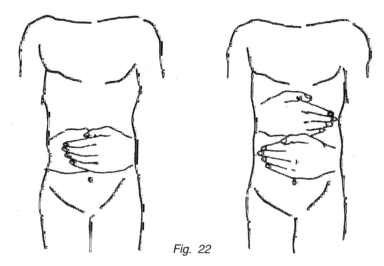

Fig. 22

17. Have the attitute of receptivity and gratitude for the Reiki energy while doing treatment either on self or others. The patient should also have the same attitude towards this energy for greater benefit.

(B) Reiki Treatment for Self

Position/ Point No.	Name of Body Part
1.	**Eyes:** Place the palms over the eyes with the fingers at the top of the forehead and the hands touching. It can be done in two ways as shown below.

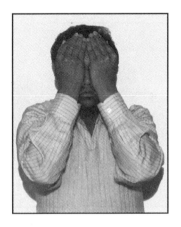 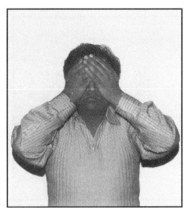

2.	**Temples**

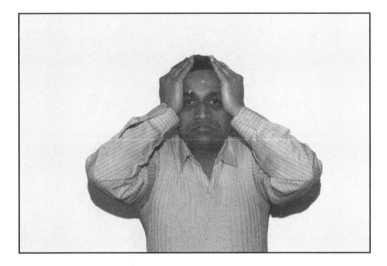

Position/ Point No.	Name of Body Part

3.   **Forehead (Ajna or Third Eye Chakra):** For giving Reiki to this point, both hands can also be placed (one over the other) on the forehead instead of one hand at front and one at the back as shown. Back Ajna Chakra can also be given Reiki separately while giving Reiki to the back side of the body (see Reiki point No. 5).

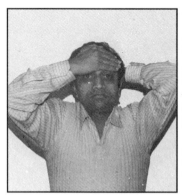 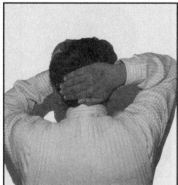

4.   **Ears:** Place the hands on the sides of the head over the ears.

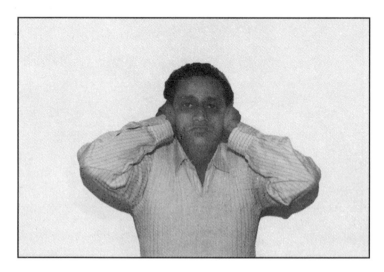

Position/ Point No.	Name of Body Part

5. **Back of Head:** Place hands on back of head with palms one over the other.

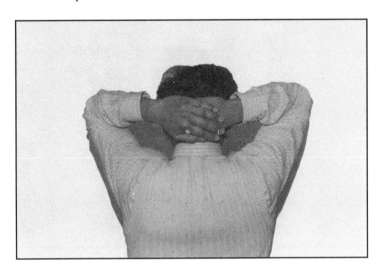

6. **Throat:** Can be done in two ways as shown.

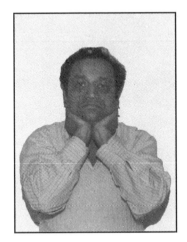 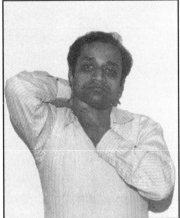

Position/ Point No.	Name of Body Part

7.   **Thymus Gland:** At collar bone level.

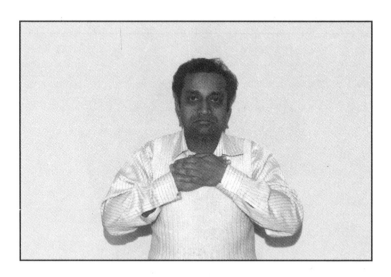

8.   **Front Heart (Anahata Chakra):** Right hand should be below left hand, i.e. right hand should touch the body. This point is located at the centre of two nipples.

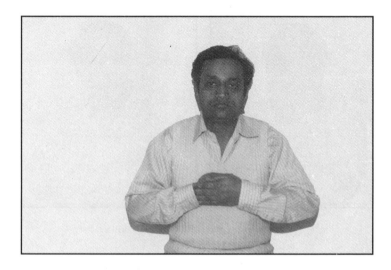

Position/	Name of Body Part
Point No.	

9.   **Front Solar Plexus (Manipura Chakra):** It is located above navel and below ribs.

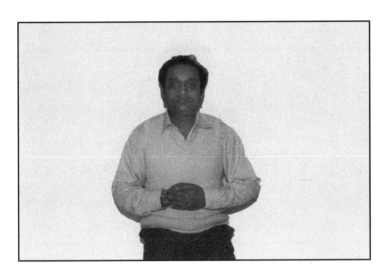

10.   **Liver and Gall Bladder:** (This point is approx. just right of solar plexus point). Hands can be put one over the other.

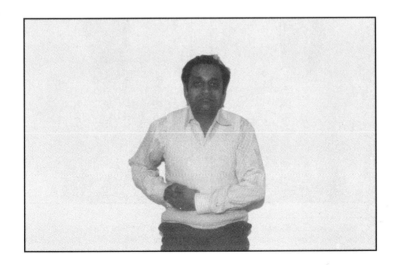

Position/ Point No.	Name of Body Part

11. **Lung Tips** (Over Clavicles)

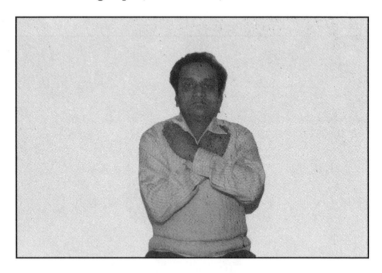

12. **Spleen and Pancreas:** (This point is just to the left of solar plexus point): Hands can be placed one over the other.

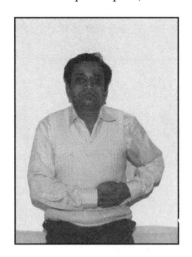 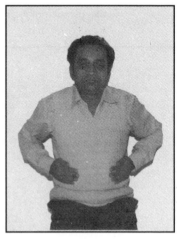

Note: Liver/Gall Bladder (Point No. 10) and Spleen/Pancreas (Point No. 12) can also be given energy simultaneously as shown above in the adjoining figure (right).

Position/ Point No.	Name of Body Part

13. **Front Hara (Swadhisthana Chakra)** : Hands to be placed below navel.

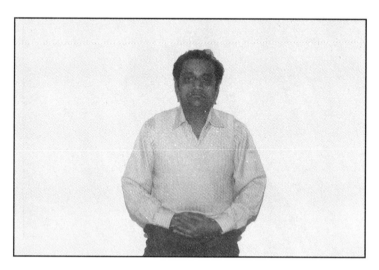

14. **Ovaries/Spermatic Cords:** Hands over the dividing line between trunk and legs (base of hands near or on hip bones, and the finger tips over the pubic bone).

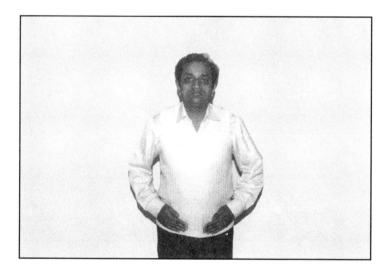

Position/ Point No.	Name of Body Part
15.	Front and Back Thigh

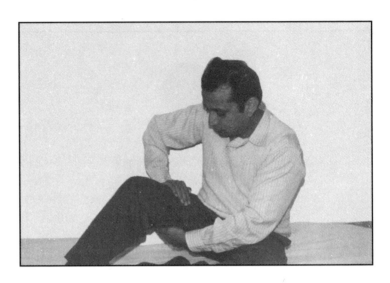

16.	Front and Back Knee

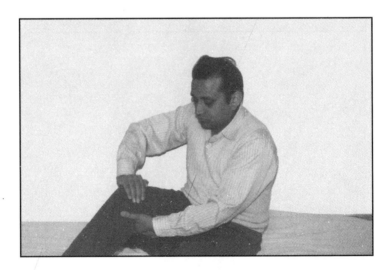

Position/ Point No.	Name of Body Part
17.	Calf

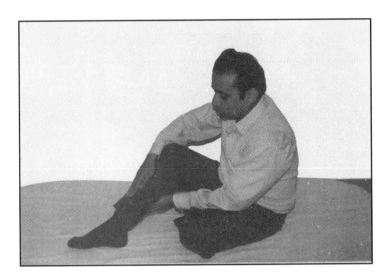

| 18. | Ankles |

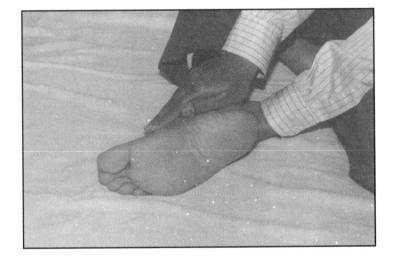

Position/ Point No.	Name of Body Part

19.   **Feet Soles:** Hold the foot with both hands–one at the sole and other on top of foot.

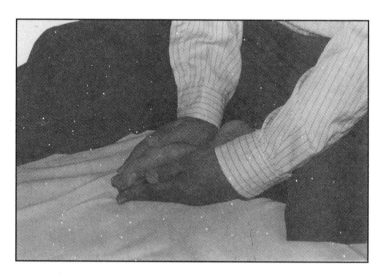

20.   **Shoulders**

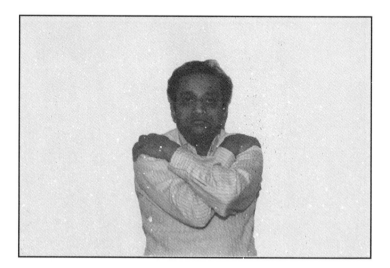

Position/ Point No.	Name of Body Part

21.   **Back Thymus:** Hands to be placed at same height as in front Thymus.

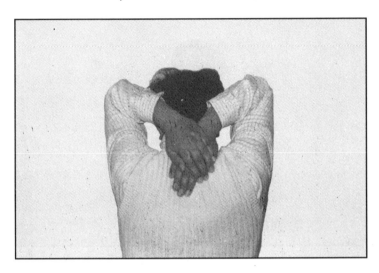

22.   **Back Heart**

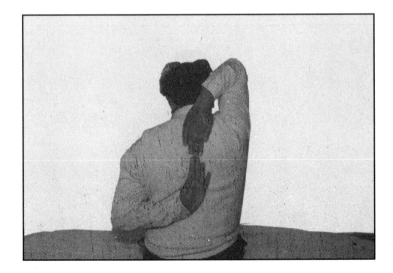

71

Position/ Point No.	Name of Body Part

23. **Back Solar Plexus:** Height same as front solar plexus.

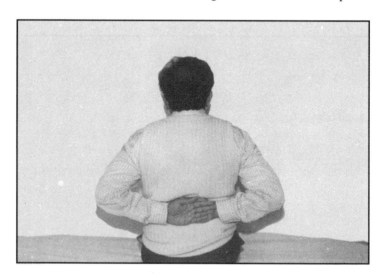

24. **Kidneys:** Level of kidneys is approx. at the level of navel, on the back of the body.

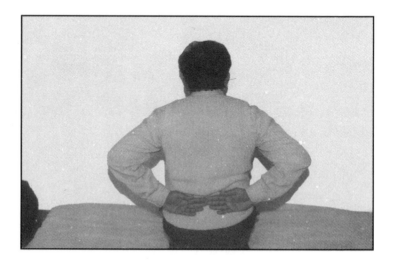

Position/ Point No.	Name of Body Part

25.   **Back Hara:** Below navel at the back of the body. Reiki at this point can also be given while lying as shown.

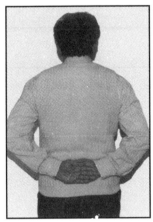 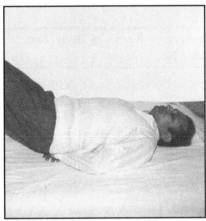

26.   **Root Chakra:** At base of spine. Reiki can also be given at this point more comfortably while lying as shown.

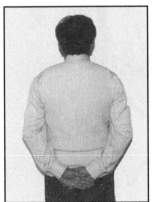 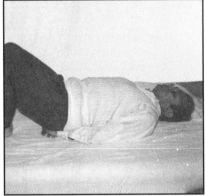

(C) Reiki Treatment for Others

Only some of the positions are shown for illustration and corresponding point nos. are mentioned. Use your intuition to give Reiki to other points on the basis of the illustrations shown.

Position/ Point No.	Name of Body Part
1.	**Eyes:** Hands are together with thumbs touching. Carefully curve the hands so that the palms do not touch the eyes or eyelashes. Slowly place the base of the hands on top of the forehead with the fingers gently resting on the cheeks. If your hands sweat, place a tissue over the eyes.

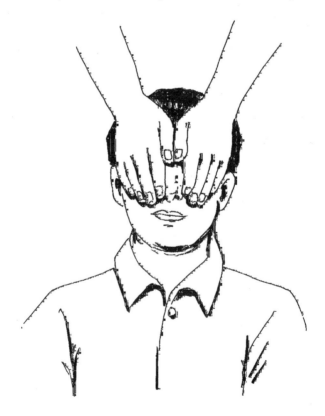

Position/ Point No.	Name of Body Part

4.   **Ears:** Place the hands on each side of the head cupped over the ears with the fingers pointing towards the feet.

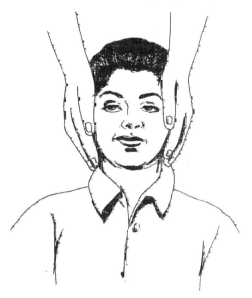

5.   **Back of Head:** Gently cradle the head in your hands. The hands are touching and the fingers are at the base of the skull.

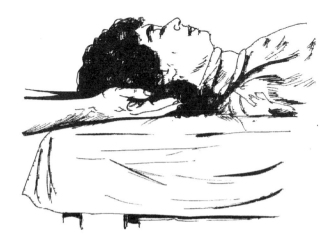

Position/ Point No.	Name of Body Part

6. **Throat:** Hands are under the chin and over the throat. One hand is over the other. Use very light pressure.

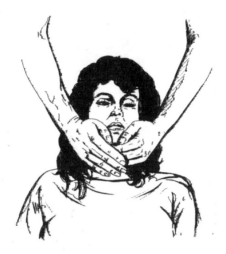

7. **Front Thymus:** Place the hands over the collar bone—one over the other.

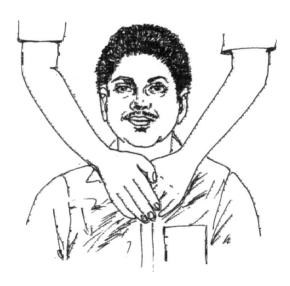

Position/ Point No.	Name of Body Part

10&12.　　**Liver/Gall Bladder** and **Spleen/Pancreas**

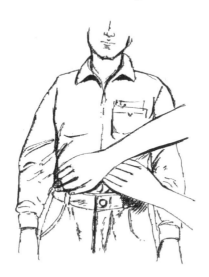

21.　　**Back Thymus**

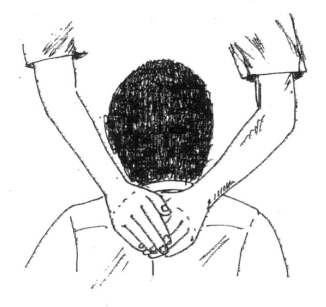

Position/ Point No.	Name of Body Part
24.	Kidneys

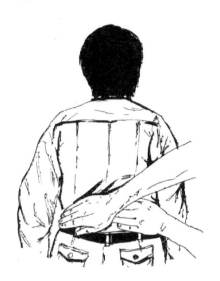

14.	Ovaries/Spermatic cords

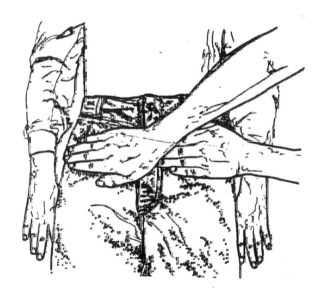

Position/ Point No.	Name of Body Part
15.	**Front Thighs:** Can change position of hands after few moments.

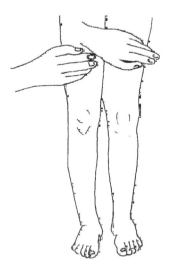

15.	**Back Thighs:** Can change position of hands after few moments.

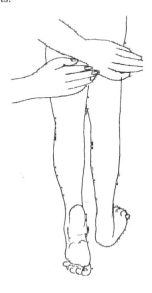

Position/ Point No.	Name of Body Part

16.   Front Knees

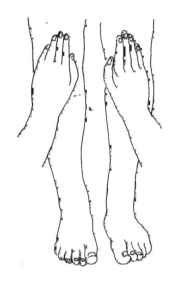

16.   Back of Knees

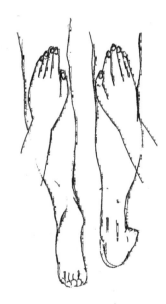

80

Position/ Point No.	Name of Body Part

17.   Back of Calves

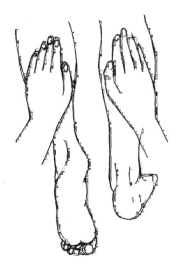

18.   **Ankles:** To be clasped from both sides.

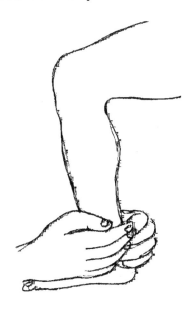

Position/ Point No.	Name of Body Part
19.	Feet and Soles

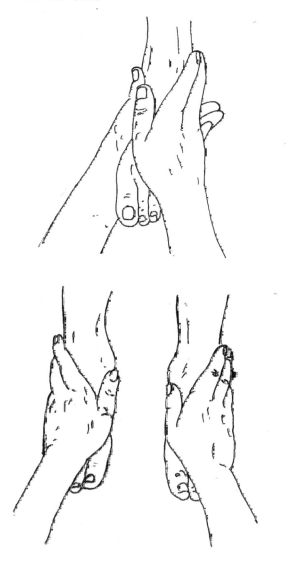

Note: In the similar way, hands can also be placed on the sole of each foot, when person is lying in prone position.

9

Reiki Treatments for Specific Ailments

(**Note:** For every treatment, Reiki Position/Point No. is given for which one can refer to chapter 8)

Sl. No.	Problem	Which part to be given Reiki	Reiki Position/ Point No.
1.	Nervous disorders, Sinusitis, Migraine, Chronic Vertigo	(a) Forehead (b) Eyes (c) Forehead and back of head (d) Temples	3 1 3 & 5 2

Note: For Migraine give Reiki on Liver also (Reiki Point No. 10).

2.	Eye problems Colour Blindness, Cataract, Glaucoma, Eye fatigue/weakness/ tiredness, etc.	Eyes	1

3.	Deafness, Hearing problem	Ears	4

4.	Cervical spondylitis spondylosis	(a) Throat both front & back (b) Back Thymus (c) Root Chakra	6 21 26

Note: One of the main causes of cervical pain is stress and unresolved emotions and inability to express & communicate themselves well.

Sl. No.	Problem	Which part to be given Reiki	Reiki Position/ Point No.
5.	Bone & muscle related problems in arms, hands, legs, feet etc.	Root Chakra	26
6.	Heart ailment, coronary artery disease, circulatory ailments, breast tumours in women	Heart Chakra	8 & 22

Note: In case of heart attack, putting right hand over back heart chakra and left hand at front solar plexus gives instant relief and takes care of emergency till patient is transported to hospital.

Sl. No.	Problem	Which part to be given Reiki	Reiki Position/ Point No.
7.	Digestive disorders, ulcers, constipation, colitis, diorrhoea	(a) Solar plexus (b) Hara	9 & 23 13
8.	Hepatitis, Jaundice Gallstones	Liver & Gall bladder	10
9.	Diabetes	(a) Hara (b) Pancreas & Spleen	13 12
10.	Fever, infections cough, cold	(a) Liver (b) Solar plexus (c) Root Chakra (d) Third Eye Chakra (both front & back)	12 9 26 3
11.	Uterian-ovarian disorders, Prostrate disorder, sexual problems	Hara	13 & 25
12.	Slipped disc, Lumbago (lower back problems)	(a) Root Chakra (b) Hara (both front & back)	26 13 & 25

Note: One of the main causes of lower back stiffness is stress & unresolved emotions.

Sl. No.	Problem	Which part to be given Reiki	Reiki Position/ Point No.
13.	General imbalance, ficklemindedness, lack of decision making in activities of life	Ankles	18
14.	Guilt and hurt feelings (which have not been reconciled & allowed to let go)	(a) Liver (b) Hara	10 13 & 25

Note: Hara is the seat of deeprooted emotions of guilt & hurt suppressed inside.

15.	Fears	(a) Root Chakra (b) Knees (c) Calves (d) Feet	26 16 17 19
16.	Anger, impatience anxiety, jealousy hatred, ego, overambition, domination, control & exploitation	(a) Solar plexus– (both front & back) (b) Back Heart (c) Hara	9 & 23 22 13 & 25
17.	Extreme nervousness, hopelessness, helplessness Causing numbness/ paralysis of limbs	(a) Back Heart (b) Thymus– (front & back) (c) Thighs– (front & back)	22 7 & 21 18

Note: Extreme hopelessness and helplessness normally causes numbness or paralysis of arms, hands & legs because arms & hands are said to be extensions of the Heart Centre which expresses love, giving & receiving. Similarly thighs are symbols of personal strength & trust. Hence giving Reiki to thighs also helps.

18.	Arthritis, rheumatism	(a) Root Chakra (b) Knees	26 16
19.	Skin problems, allergies	(a) Spleen (b) Liver (c) Root Chakra	12 10 26

Sl. No.	Problem	Which part to be given Reiki	Reiki Position/ Point No.
20.	Kidney related problems, urinary problems	(a) Kidneys (b) Root Chakra (c) Hara	24 26 13 & 25
21.	Growth disorder, lack of general vitality & stamina, general weakness & fatigue	(a) Root Chakra (b) Sole Chakra	26 19
22.	Shoulder pain	Shoulders	20

Note: Many of cervical & shoulder pains arise due to psychological causes of taking excessive personal or other's responsibilities and their emotional & mental burdens.

Sl. No.	Problem	Which part to be given Reiki	Reiki Position/ Point No.
23.	Cramps & stiffness in calves	(a) Kness (b) Calves (c) Feet (d) Thighs	6 17 19 15

Note: The psychological reason for cramps & stiffness in calves is resistance to changes and inability to move forward in life.

Sl. No.	Problem	Which part to be given Reiki	Reiki Position/ Point No.
24.	High blood pressure	(a) Solar plexus (b) Hara (c) Kidneys (d) Root	9 & 23 13 & 25 24 26
25.	Insomnia	(a) Place right hand on front heart & Left hand on front Hara (b) Ears (c) Third Eye Chakra	8 & 13 4 3
26.	Upper back stiffness and rigidity	(a) Back Thymus (b) Shoulders (c) Throat	21 20 6

Note: One of the main causes of upper back stiffness is stress and unresolved/repressed emotions.

Sl. No.	Problem	Which part to be given Reiki	Reiki Position/ Point No.
27.	Asthma	(a) Solar Plexus (b) Back Heart (c) Throat	9 22 6

10

Distant Healing

It is also possible to send Reiki across space and do distant or absent healing. As explained earlier, life energy or prana is semiphysical in nature, that is, it has properties both of physical and non-physical nature. It is this non-physical nature which enables it to be sent across space.

To send Reiki to someone at a distance you have to first visualize him in your mind's eye. The better the visualization the better the energy transmission. If you want to treat a specific area or organ of someone's body then visualize that area. When you are calm and relaxed, visualization is better. Hence it is better to first calm and centre yourself by focussing on some neutral thing like your own breathing or some visual focus or some background soothing sound.

After visualization of the healee or his specific area, imagine that you are giving/beaming Reiki to him by your hands just as you will give when he is physically present with you. For better visualization of transfer of energy, you may also pose your hands as if you are physically focussing Reiki on the visualized area. In fact, by using the imagination to bring into mind a strong clear picture of the other person, you induce an en-rapport condition in which he will be practically in the same psychic relation to you as if he were actually before you. If the healee also focuses upon you at that time (if you inform him beforehand when you will be giving healing to him), the results will be still better. Hence in distant healing, the strong concentration of healer in healing (so as not to lose visualization) plays a vital role unlike touch healing where too much focus or concentration is not needed. There are other advanced methods also for giving distant healing by using symbols etc which are outside the scope of this book.

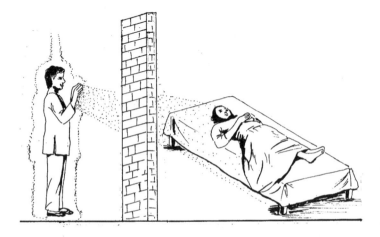

Fig. 23: Visualizing Beaming Reiki to a Distant Person

11

Scanning and Treating The Aura

*(**Note:** Most of the material and figures in this chapter have been taken from Master Choa Kok Sui's famous book "Miracles through Pranic Healing", Chapter 3 titled 'Elementary Pranic Healing'. We convey our heartfelt gratitude to them).*

Scanning and healing the energy field or aura is very healthy. The cause of most illnesses and other problems is usually in the aura. By treating the aura, you will be working on the cause and also will be healing problems before they get a chance to develop in the physical body. Also, once a problem develops in the body, the problem in the aura can become worse. In addition, healing the aura first, helps the person's energy field accept Reiki more completely and allows it to flow more easily where it is needed when giving a regular Reiki treatment. Therefore, if you are going to do both scanning and a regular Reiki treatment, scanning should be done first.

Hands Sensitization for Scanning

The attunement process not only opens the palm chakras so that Reiki can flow, it also heigtens their sensitivity to Pranic energy. Further, sensitivity can be increased by following the measures given in chapter 7. By using the chakras in the palms of your hands, it is possible to scan the aura of client and locate the diseased areas in bioplasmic body.

Process of Scanning the Aura

Place your left hand (or non-dominant hand) about 12" away from the top of the person's head. Place your consciousness in the palm of your hand and notice how it feels. Then move your hand closer to about 3–4" from the top of the head and begin moving your hand over the person's face and moving down toward the feet continuing to remain about 3–4" away from the body. Move your hand very slowly and be aware of any changes in the energy feeling on the palm of your hand.

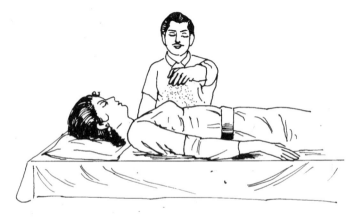

Fig. 24: Scanning the Aura

When you feel any change at all, then you will know that this is a place where the person needs Reiki. You may feel coolness, warmth, tingling, pressure, little electric shocks, pulsations, distortion, irregularity or a pulling. The change may be very slight and you may think it is your imagination. However, trust in your experience. Remember, when you first begin to practise scanning, your sensitivity may not be that much developed, so you need to pay very close attention. As you practise, your ability to scan the body will improve. After a while, you may even find that you can scan with your eyes and sense where the problems are, or you could begin to actually see the distressed areas.

Interpretation of Results of Scanning the Aura

While scanning the aura, you may find two types of pranic imbalances at specific portions of the body.

(A) Pranic Depletion

These are areas where you will notice hollows in the client's aura. The affected part is depleted of prana. The surrounding fine meridians are partially or severely blocked preventing fresh prana from other parts to flow freely and vitalize the affected part. Therefore affected part or chakra is depleted and filled with dirty diseased bioplasmic matter and becomes partly inactivated.

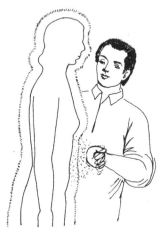

Fig. 25: Pranic Depletion

(B) Pranic Congestion

These are areas where you will find protrusions in the client's aura indicating pranic congestion in these parts. This also causes the surrounding fine meridians to be partially or severely blocked. This congested prana and bioplasmic matter can't flow freely and hence becomes diseased after a certain period of time since fresh prana can't flow in properly. The affected chakra is congested and filled with diseased bioplasmic matter.

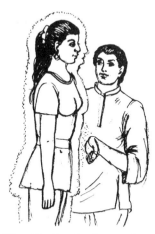

Fig. 26: Pranic Congestion

It may be noted that more the hollow or protrusion in the health aura, more severe is the sickness.

Healing the Aura

As soon as you find a change in the energy field while scanning the aura, move your hand up and down until you find the height where you feel the most distortion. This could be as high as several feet above the body or you may feel compelled to actually touch the body with your hands.

When you find the right height, bring both hands together at this spot and channel Reiki. Reiki will heal the problem in the aura and also flow into the physical body and work on the organs and tissues connected to the problems in the aura.

Remain channeling Reiki at the detected spot until you feel the flow of Reiki subsiding or until you feel the area is healed. Then re-scan the area to confirm that it is healed–if not, you can continue to give Reiki there until it feels complete. Then move your hand down along the length of body until you find another area in need of healing and do Reiki there. Continue until you have scanned and healed the whole energy field.

Self-scanning

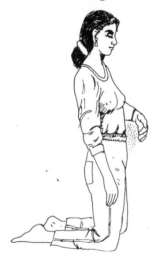

Fig. 27 Self-scanning

The scanning process can also be done on yourself. Follow the same steps as above, looking for distortions and administering Reiki when you find them.

In addition to scanning the aura and treating it by giving Reiki, one should also ponder over the causes of distortion of energy at those particular places by looking into one's lifestyle and personal problems being faced and then try to remove those root causes by proper integration of your personality.

Cleansing the Aura by Sweeping

Sweeping is generally an aura cleansing technique and it serves the following purposes: (Fig. 28)

(a) It removes congested and diseased bioplasmic matter from energy body. Blocked meridians and bioplasmic channels are thus opened. This allows prana from other parts of the body to flow to the affected part.

(b) To distribute excess prana from one part to other.

(c) It seals holes in the aura through which prana leaks out.

(d) Health rays are properly combed and strengthened and the resulting strong health aura acts as a protective shield, increases one's resistance against infection.

There are two hand positions in sweeping:

(i) Cupped hand position: It is mostly used to remove the diseased bioplasmic matter.

(ii) Spread finger position: It is more effective in combing and strengthening health rays.

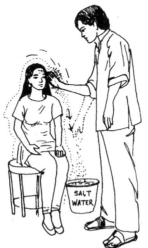

Fig. 28: Localized Sweeping

93

Sweeping is of two types:

(i) *General sweeping*: when cleansing is done on the whole bioplasmic body.

(ii) *Localized sweeping*: When cleansing is done on specific parts of the body.

Process of Local Sweeping

Place your hands just above the affected area. Then with proper concentration, sweep away the diseased bioplasmic matter with quick back-forth circular movement of cupped hand and then strongly flick your hand in salt water kept in a bowl. Do it 20 to 30 times. This is very useful in case of local pains like headache, etc.

Process of General Sweeping

General sweeping is done with a series of downward sweeping movements. You start from the head down to the feet. Maintain a distance of about 2" from the patient's body to

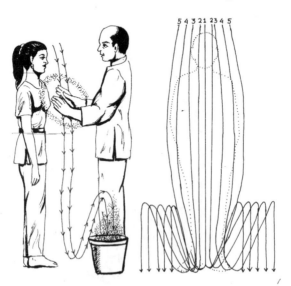

Fig. 29: General Sweeping

94

your hands. With your hands cupped, sweep your hands slowly downward from the head to the foot following line no. 1 in the figure. Then slightly raise your hands and strongly flick them in a salt water unit to throw away the diseased energy. It is very important. Now repeat the same procedure with spread finger position to comb and strengthen the health rays. Now repeat the whole process on lines 2, 3, 4 & 5. Downward sweeping can be applied both on front and back of body. Repeat this process few times.

General sweeping can be done with patient standing, sitting or lying down. This technique is very effective in treating conditions where the whole body appears to be filled with diseased energy, e.g. fever, cancer, multiple diseases in body, degeneration of multiple joints, muscles, bones etc.

Protecting the Aura

There are certain circumstances in which it is both permissible and desirable to form either a shell or shield of etheric (or pranic) matter to protect oneself from unpleasant influences of various kinds.

For example, in a mixed crowd there is quite likely to be present etheric vibrations which are distasteful and injurious. Or again, it may be necessary to sleep e.g. in a railway carriage in close proximity with people of the vampire type or whose emanations are coarse and undesirable; or one may have to visit persons or places where disease is rampant. Similarly places like burial sites, crematorium, market places, railway stations may be possible examples of negative energy.

In all these cases, an etheric shell may be utilized with advantage to protect oneself. It is important to note, however, that an etheric shell which keeps away outside etheric matter will also keep your etheric matter in and that therefore one's own etheric emanations, many of which are poisonous, will also be kept within the shell.

Hence etheric shield should be made only where you feel that outside atmosphere is filled with more of negative energy than positive. If you continue to maintain etheric shield even at the place which is filled with positive energy then you will be deprived of valuable positive energy which helps in diluting or throwing your negative energy and adding positive to it.

The protective shield is made simply by an effort of will and imagination where you mentally affirm and visualize that *'I am surrounded by a strong etheric shield which will reflect away all the negative vibrations coming to it. I deny the entry of any negative vibrations in my aura'.* In this positive statement you have the occult shield of defence which is a mighty protection to you. It will be better to reaffirm this visualization frequently so as to reinforce it. For shielding, some people visualize themselves surrounded by purple colour mirrored boxes which will reflect back the outside and inside vibrations and won't allow them to pass. You may also shield your home, office or car in the same manner. At the appropriate time, when shield is no more needed, i.e. when you are no more in the atmosphere of negative or mixed up vibrations, again visualize the shield to disappear.

12

Supporting Aids for Reiki Practice

While you are practising Reiki, you should also ensure that your lifestyle is such which keeps your energy body clean, positive and strong. This will be very favourable to your Reiki healing practices. We are giving below some of the measures which will help in keeping your energy body pure and strong:

1. Refrain from eating meat. Such foods contain lot of toxins secreted by animal during killing. Moreover, meat is considered Tamsik food with lot of negative energy.

2. Do occasional fasting with water and fruit juices. It will keep your system clean.

3. Stop or minimize caffeine drinks (e.g. coffee, tea, soft drinks, chocolate etc.). They create imbalance in the nervous and endocrine system and hence in the energy body.

4. Stop alcohol intake.

5. Minimize taking sweets and white sugar products.

6. Stop or minimize smoking.

7. Relax and meditate regularly. Sitting postures of meditation (with straight spine) help a lot for balancing your pranic flow in the body. See Fig. 30.

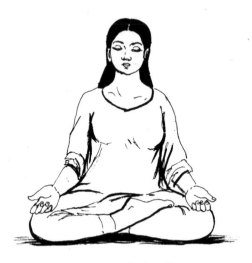

Fig. 30: Meditation Posture

8. Reduce time in watching TV, listening to Radio, reading newspapers and stray magazines. Excessive involvement in these things distract the mind and thereby affect the balance of energy body.

9. Go for regular walks in morning/evening in fresh air. Do moderate exercises and yogasanas with special emphasis on spinal exercises to keep it supple and straight. See Fig. 31.

   Note: To understand more about anatomy of spine and exercises to keep it healthy, refer my book, **'Freedom from Cervical and Back Pain.**

10. Drink water stored in gold, silver or copper vessels. Water charged with these metals becomes filled with positive energy. Magnetized water is equally good.

11. Do pranayama or breathing exercises. They are very effective in balancing and strengthening your energy field. Specially develop the habit of rhythmic and diaphragmatic breathing as your moment to moment resting breathing. It has a very benevolent effect in maintaining a healthy aura. See Fig. 32.

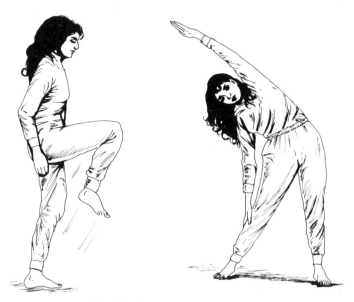

Fig. 31: Yogasanas and Exercises

12. Spend time with nature whenever you get opportunity. Take sunbath in the morning. Fire element of our body is easily rejuvenated by sunbath.

13. Have regular water bath and do friction rubbing of body either by hand or by bath brush before bathing. Bathing in flowing river water is very good. Occasional bathing with salt water helps in cleansing the negative energy as salt has the characteristic of breaking down the negative energy. Among salts, sea salt is said to be especially useful.

Some people do foot soaking in salt water. Water can be lukewarm, hot or cold depending upon your body's demand at a particular time. This is a very effective method for removing the negative energy of the body through the feet which is sucked by salt water. After foot soaking, this water should be thrown into W.C. because this water becomes impure after absorbing negativity.

Foot soaking in salt water is said to clear our Swadhisthana and solar plexus chakra.

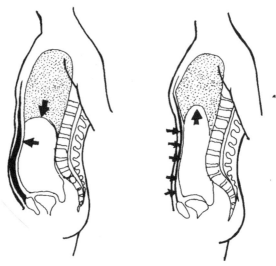

Fig. 32: Diaphragmatic Breathing

During inhalation the diaphragm contracts downwards and the abdomen expands

During exhalation the diaphragm relaxes abdomen contracts

14. Walk barefoot on earth specially near river and countryside and on grass wet with morning dew. The earth element sucks lot of negativity through our feet and clears our Mooladhara chakra (or Root chakra). Sole chakra is an extension of Root chakra and is related directly to it. Sole chakra is also said to be related to Heart chakra.

15. Increase your awareness and attention in every task you do. This will increase your power and sensitivity to sense subtle impressions and sensations within and around you.

16. Laugh a lot. Laughing is a potent medicine for supplying you with instant positive energy. If you find difficult to laugh in your normal life routine, then read jokes in magazines/books, see comedy serials on TV, read entertainment columns of magazines etc. Also develop the habit of cutting and hearing jokes frequently (within limits of decency). Try to wear a natural smile on your face. This will keep you effortlessly positive.

17. Be aware of negative emotions (e.g. anger, fear, jealousy, hate, worry, impatience, hurry, revenge, etc.). Whenever they are arising in you, nip them in the bud at the very outset. Negative emotions throw your energy body completely out of balance.

18. After practising any energy gathering techniques in the body, sit for sometime by joining fingers of both hands together (see fig. 33). This conserves and

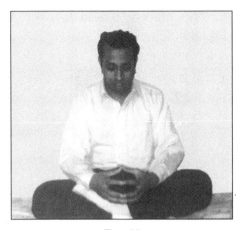

Fig. 33

harmonizes the energy flow on both sides of body and doesn't allow energy to dissipate outside.

19. Take some measures for keeping your home and work environment clean for creating a positive energy field as mentioned below:

(i) Evaporate pure camphor crystals. An easy way to do it is with the help of an electronic mosquito repellent. Place the camphor on a used mat. This way the camphor evaporates very slowly over many hours.

(ii) Burn incense ('Agarbatti's and 'Dhoops'). Their smell also purifies the energy of the surroundings.

(iii) Following oils have the power to create positive energy and neutralize negative energy. Hence burn oil lamp of the following oils:

(a) Mustard oil

(b) Sesame (Til) oil

(c) Ghee or clarified butter

(iv) Candle burning also neutralizes negative energy and creates positive energy. 'Trataka' on candle flame is very good because its light clears out the negative energy. This practice is said to clear Ajna Chakra. (See Fig. 34).

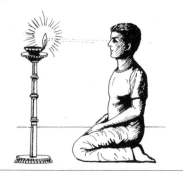

Fig. 34: Oil Lamp Creates Positive Energy

(v) Salt water specially sea-salt water has great potential for neutralizing negative energy. One can mop the floor with sea-salt water or one can even keep a bowl of sea-salt water in a corner of the room. Every now and then put the bowl in the sun for a few hours and top it up and also change the water completely after certain days.

(vi) Fresh cut flowers with leaves and stems intact, placed in water in a vase or bowl and indoor plants are great positive energy generators and negative energy neutralizers. Yellow, orange and blue/violet flowers are quite good for this purpose.

(vii) Use those colours in your surroundings (room walls, curtains, carpet, furniture, wearing clothes) which promote positive energy and transmute negative energy. Such colours are white, blue-violet, green, yellow, orange, rose etc. Even visualizing these colours in meditation helps you in getting their positive energy.

(viii) Just like colours, there are certain sounds which generate positive energy and transmute negative energy. All Satwik sounds and music come under this category. These sounds are found generally in old melodious songs and music, devotional songs, soul stirring bhajans, classical music, flute music, sound vibrations generated by blowing into a conch-shell ('Shankh') and sounds simulating nature sounds e.g. sound of waterfall, flowing river, moving breeze, chirping of birds etc. By listening to such sounds, you always feel calm, centred, joyful and elevated. On the other hand, the modern Rajasik music like pop music only gives momentary thrill and excitement and hence it is not good for energy body.

(ix) Foodgrains, specially rice (uncooked), have the capacity to absorb and transmute negative energies. In particular, on the eleventh day of the waxing and waning moon cycle, this absorption is at a maximum. This day is called 'Ekadasi' (eleventh day). Hence they are kept in 'Pooja' (worship) places.

(x) Chanting of Mantras and *Nama-Japa* creates an energy pure environment mainly because of effect of satwik sound vibrations. However, mental japa of mantras is equally effective in purifying the environment because the pure thought vibrations created by mental japa also act on the energy atmosphere around because of the relationship between thought and life energy.

(xi) Tulsi leaves are very effective in destroying the negative energy and purifying the atmosphere by creating positive energy. Hence always keep Tulsi plants in your terrace/balcony.

The positive energy atmosphere thus generated by the above measures will tend to neutralize negative energy in your energy body and increase positive energy. These two processes of decrease in negative energy and increase in positive energy happen simultaneously in your energy body whenever any positive energy is supplied to you. Hence these two processes are interrelated and not independent of each other. However, some of these measures only neutralize or break down negative energy without supplying additional positive energy, e.g. salt water treatment, uncooked rice treatment etc.

13

Balancing Panch Pranas

Our ancient yoga literature have talked about five kinds of prana (or life energy). Thus, vitality or life energy flows through the body in five main streams (though there are many subdivisions). Each prana is located in a different region of the body and regulates the health of the parts of the body of that region. These five types of prana or life energy are associated with five elements and five chakras (below Ajna chakra). The following table shows these correspondences and their functions in the body.

Sl. No.	Name of Prana	Region/ Location	Chakra	Corres- ponding Sense	Element	Colour	Function
1.	Prana	Heart	Anahata (Heart)	Touch	Air	Green	Respiration
2.	Apana	Anus	Root	Smell	Earth	Red	Excretion
3.	Samana	Navel	Solar Plexus	Sight	Fire	Yellow	Digestion
4.	Udana	Throat	Vishuddhi	Hearing	Ether (or Akasa/ sky/empty space)	Blue	Swallowing, facial expression, speech
5.	Vyana	Entire body	Hara/ spleen	Taste	Water	Red- orange/ Rose	Blood circul- ation, nervous system

Now the five elements corresponding to five pranas mentioned above are represented in our hands as shown below:

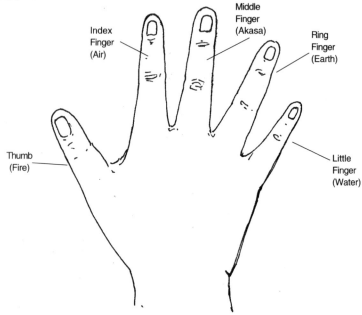

Fig. 35: Five Elements Represented in Five Fingers

Imbalance of these pranas or elements in the body causes diseases in the body. Indian sages discovered that by joining different fingers and thumbs in specific ways, all these elements and pranas are brought into balance and diseases connected with their imbalances are cured. This was named as 'Mudra Vigyan' or Science of Postures.

We give below the details of such mudras, and advise you to practise them in addition to Reiki healing for further balancing and strengthening of your life energy flow.

Which Element is Active at a Particular Time

Condition of elements in the body can be told by yogis through the principles of Swara Yoga. In Swara Yoga, by analyzing the breath from nostrils, one finds out which 'Tattwa' or element is active because at one time one 'Tattwa' is more active compared to others. Since every element corresponds to a particular chakra, hence it can be known which prana and chakra is more active. Each tattwa produces different types of exhaled breath causing the air to flow out from different points of the nostrils in a particular direction and extending to a certain distance. For example, following patterns are observed:

(1) When Earth element is active, breath (exhalation) flows from the center, going straight forward.

(2) Water element makes the breath flow slightly downward, leaving the nostrils from the lower point.

(3) Fire element makes the breath flow from the upper point in an upward direction.

(4) Air element makes the breath flow predominantly from the outer sides and breath can be felt moving at an angle.

(5) When Ether (or Akasa) is active, it will seem that there is no exhalation escaping, only the warmth of the hot air will be felt on hand.

Another way to find the active 'tattwa' is to judge the vapour pattern formed by exhaling through the nose into a mirror

(a) If vapour covers the mirror, earth is active.

(b) A half moon shape indicates water.

(c) A triangular shape indicates fire.

(d) An egg or oval shape indicates air.

(e) Small dots indicate ether.

So by studying which Tattwa is active a person can get a clue about the flow of a particular type of prana and activity of the corresponding chakra and take corrective action if required in line with the activity of that prana and chakra.

Sl. No.	Name & Description of Mudra	Benefits
1.	**Gyan Mudra:** Touch the tip of thumb with tip of index finger. 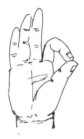 *Fig. 36*	Increases concentration, brain power, memory. Cures insomnia, tensions and various mental ailments.
2.	**Vayu Mudra (Air):** Put the index finger at the base of thumb and press it lightly with thumb. 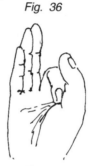 *Fig. 37*	·Cures rheumatism, gout, arthritis, Parkinson's disease, blood circulation defects, gas and indigestion.
3.	**Shunya Mudra (Space):** Put the middle finger at the base of thumb on mount of Venus and press it lightly with thumb. 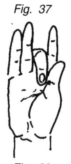 *Fig. 38*	Cures earache, deafness, vertigo.
4.	**Prithvi Mudra (Earth):** Touch the tip of ring finger with the tip of thumb. Keep other fingers straight. 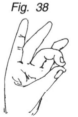 *Fig. 39*	Cures weakness of body and makes the body robust, sturdy and full of vigour.

108

Sl. No.	Name & Description of Mudra		Benefits
5.	**Varun Mudra (Water):** Touch the tip of little finger with tip of thumb.	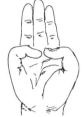 *Fig. 40*	Cures impurities of blood, skin problems. Useful in gastro-enteritis and any other disease causing dehydration.
6.	**Sun Mudra:** Put ring finger at the base of thumb and press that finger lightly with thumb.	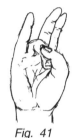 *Fig. 41*	It creates heat in body, helps in digestion and in reducing fat in the body.
7.	**Pran Mudra:** Touch the tips of little and ring fingers with the tip of thumb.	 *Fig. 42*	It increases life force and cures fatigue. Imparts special power to the eyes.
8.	**Ling Mudra:** Interlock the fingers of both the hands with palms joined together. Keep the left thumb upright encircled with the right thumb and right index finger.	 *Fig. 43*	It creates heat in the body and cures cold, cough, bronchial infections. It increases the general resistance power of body against changes in weather, fever, infections, etc.

Sl. No.	Name & Description of Mudra	Benefits

9. **Apaan Mudra:** Lightly touch the tips of second and third fingers with the tip of thumb.

Fig. 44

Helps in elimination of waste matter from mouth, eyes, ears, nose and other excretory organs etc. Reduces constipation. Helps in stomach ache also.

10. **Apaan Vayu Mudra:** It is a combination of Apaan and Vayu Mudra.

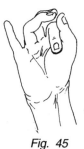

Fig. 45

Good for heart ailments. Acts as first aid for heart attack. Reduces palpitation

11. **Vyana Mudra:** Join the tips of index and middle fingers with the tip of thumb.

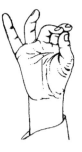

Fig. 46

Controls blood pressure.

14

Energy Locks

They are also called 'Bandhas' in the language of Yoga. They are special postures adopted to conserve and make use of vast reserve of prana. They not only prevent dissipation of prana but also enable you to regulate its flow and convert it into spiritual energy. They are said to raise the latent Kundalini energy by their powerful effect on flow of prana. Along with Reiki, practising these techniques will help you further in strengthening your energy body. Of course, your other yoga practices like asana, pranayama, meditation, vegetarian diet, etc. should continue for added benefits.

There are mainly three kinds of 'Bandhas' or 'Locks' as described below:

(1) *Jalandhar Bandha:* While retaining your breath after inhaling, press your chin firmly into the chest. This prevents 'prana' escaping from upper body. Lift your head while you exhale. (Fig. 47, next page)

By pressing the chin against the chest, carotid arteries in the neck are pressed reducing the blood flow into brain resulting in a state akin to artificial anaesthesia or trance.

(2) *Uddiyana Bandha:* After exhaling completely, pull the abdomen up and back towards the spine as much

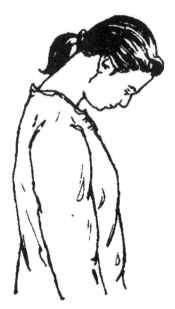

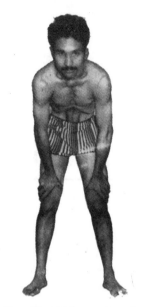

Fig. 47: Jalandhar Bandha   Fig. 48: Uddiyana Bandha

as possible. This forces Prana-Apana up the Sushumna Nadi. (See Fig. 48)

(3) Moola Bandha: While retaining the breath, contract the anal sphincter muscles. This prevents the apana escaping from the lower body and helps in drawing it up to unite with prana.

15

Kundalini and Reiki

Many people remain confused about the relationship of Kundalini energy with Reiki. On the basis of my extensive study whatever little I have understood in this regard, I am sharing it with the readers.

Kundalini is also the source of life energy. Difference between the energy of Reiki and Kundalini is that while Reiki comes from the above (top, Crown Chakra), Kundalini energy rises from below. At the stage of enlightenment both these energies meet or fuse into each other. In fact, during enlightenment by Kundalini awakening, Kundalini reaches to Sahasrara Chakra and merges into Universal life energy. Similarly we can achieve enlightenment by taking Reiki down to meet Kundalini. End results are same by both the processes.

In an ordinary person only the grosser aspect of Kundalini energy is working through 'Ida' and 'Pingala' nadis which serves to fulfill only bodily needs. However the inner aspect of Kundalini which works through Sushumna nadi remains dormant. Or even if it is opened, it is opened only up to the level of lower three chakras. But very small energy is going to the higher chakras through the Sushumna nadi. This inner aspect of Kundalini is associated with our level of consciousness and spiritual development. However, when Kundalini is fully awakened, all the energy starts flowing through Sushumna and we attain higher levels of consciousness and then everything is looked and understood from a higher level of awareness. Energywise also, body receives full and balanced energy when energy is following through Sushumna instead of Ida and Pingala.

Some schools of occultism believe that life energy is bipolar in nature, i.e. it is made up of both male and female healing energies. The male part comes from above and is associated with Reiki and Crown Chakra. The female part comes from below and is associated with Kundalini and Root Chakra. These two energies communicate with each other and decide how much of each polarity is needed.

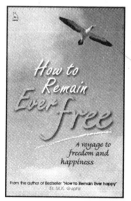

How to Remain Ever Free is a masterpiece by the well-known author of self-management books, Er. M.K. Gupta. This book has a vibe and style of its own which makes it completely different from the other books of this category. Once in hand, the reader flows effortlessly with the book feeling continuously the presence and vibrations of the author.

In this book, the author takes you on a journey towards freedom and happiness. According to him, freedom is the very fragrance of life. Freedom and happiness are very intimately linked with each other. However, the author makes a clear distinction between real freedom and the so called casual freedom of doing anything as per one's whims and fancies. In real freedom, one remains a master while in casual or apparent freedom, you are actually a slave or servant, though outwardly, you may appear wearing the mask of freedom.

In the present book, the author gives various tips on freedom from various negative and undesirable traits from your personality. Once negativities disappear from your being, what remains is only positivity which will give you nothing but happiness. According to the author, every human being has got both Lower and Higher nature in his being. When we fall towards our Lower nature, we are going towards slavery and unhappiness. Similarly, when we rise in our Higher nature, we are going towards freedom and happiness. All our negativities are a part of our Lower nature while all our positive qualities are part of our Higher nature.

Like, the author's earlier book, *How to Remain Ever Happy*, this book too is divided into small chapters with pleasing illustrations to avoid monotony while reading the book. Further, you can read the book from anywhere as every chapter is independent and complete in itself.

Demy size • Pages: 208 • Price: Rs. 96/- • Postage: Rs. 15/-

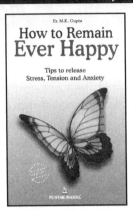

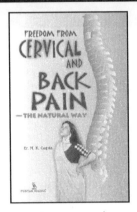

How to Remain Ever Happy

'How to Remain Ever Happy' is a masterpiece by the famous author of self-management books Er. M.K. Gupta, giving you countless practical tips for enjoying happiness in your day to day life.

The notable feature of the book is that you can start reading from any page as every tip is complete and independent in itself.

The author gives a message in short one or two page tips, which eliminates completely the scope of boredom or monotony. You will feel like flowing effortlessly with the matter while reading the book. Over 120 tips to make your life brighter and happier!

(also available in Hindi & Bangla)

Demy Size • Pages: 168
Price: Rs. 96/- • Postage: Rs. 15/-

Freedom from Cervical and Back Pain

Two of the most incapacitating ailments in modern times are cervical pain and backache. Both ailments can severely hamper a person's movement, denting the patient's personal and professional life. There is no permanent cure in allopathy for both ailments. Painkillers and other medications simply provide temporary relief... until the next spasm of excruciating pain shoots through the body again.

The book puts all relevant issues regarding the two ailments in proper perspective. At the outset, it highlights the proper postures that can help prevent backache and cervical pain. It also lists the precautions to be taken while exercising. Patients are then taught how to find relief through the practice of Yoga. If practised regularly with patience and diligence, Yoga can provide permanent relief to patients. The book tells readers how to maintain good posture and perform loosening and strengthening exercises for the muscles that gradually restore the tone and alignment of these muscles before degenerative and irreversible damage occurs.

Demy Size • Pages: 128
Price: Rs. 80/- • Postage: Rs. 15/-

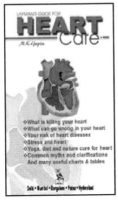

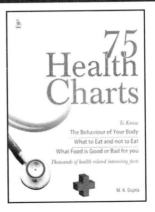

Layman's Guide for Heart Care

In simple terms, the book outlines the working of the human heart, the factors that affect it and what can go wrong. It also helps the reader gauge where he or she stands vis-à-vis heart disease. The diagnoses and various types of heart disease are dealt with subsequently. A variety of risk factors are also highlighted. These include stress, smoking and alcohol, faulty diet, obesity, sedentary lifestyles, blood pressure and diabetes, among others.

The subsequent chapters dwell on the medical treatments for heart ailments. Besides modern medical techniques, the book also tells readers about non-invasive and natural methods such as Yoga and other nature-cure alternatives.

In conclusion, the book dispels common myths surrounding this modern killer disease and enlightens readers on the true facts. Peppered with many useful charts, tables and illustrations, the book can serve as a handy guide for those suffering from heart disease or as a preventive manual for those with a family history of heart ailments.

Demy Size • Pages: 120
Price: Rs. 80/- • Postage: Rs. 15/-

75 Health Charts

As any health-conscious person knows, health is truly wealth. Yet, simply harbouring good intentions does not ensure good health for anyone. Beginning in infancy and right up to our twilight years, a conscious attempt has to be made to lead a healthy lifestyle. In the formative years, our parents make this effort on our behalf. But as we enter the teens and take control of our own destinies, how well informed we are on health-related issues makes all the difference between physical well-being and ill health.

This book ensures you have all the facts, figures and data at your fingertips to promote proper health and nutrition in order to prevent disease.

In this book you will find: height and weight charts, blood pressure and pulse rate charts, calorie charts, fat and cholesterol charts, vitamin and mineral charts, balanced diet charts, pollution health hazard charts, infectious diseases and immunisation charts, healthy heart and stress charts... not to mention other relevant charts, tables and data.

Big Size • Pages: 144
Price: Rs. 120/- • Postage: Rs. 15/-

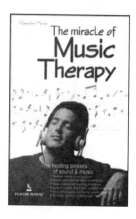

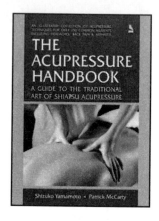

The Miracle of Music Therapy

—Rajendar Menen

Music is all around us. It marks every event of our life, from birth, marriage and death to the phases in-between. Man has long known that music has the ability to calm, cajole and rejuvenate. But it is only recently that science has begun to understand, study and document the effects of music in methodology, which leaves little room for doubt.

It is now an established fact that music helps all living creatures—from plants to birds and animals and man—to grow and rejuvenate. Music permeates the cells of all living beings, alters mood swings, cell division, heals the ailing.

While the *rishis* of ancient India and the Vedas first documented the effects of music on the human beings and all living things, it was left to the western world to fashion the more modern concepts of healing through music. This book dwells heavily on the findings from ancient India and the masters of today who have made music therapy a viable healing alternative. It is the most comprehensive guide on the healing powers of sound and music.

Demy Size • Pages: 144
Price: Rs. 80/- • Postage: Rs. 15/-

The Acupressure Handbook

A guide to the traditional art of Shiatsu Acupressure

—Shizuko Yamamoto & Patrick McCarty

This unique book is a comprehensive collection of acupressure techniques and natural healing remedies designed to bring about immediate relief from a variety of pains and illnesses. Using easy-to-follow instructions and numerous photographs and illustrations, this book guides you through the various applications of *Shiatsu* massage.

This book is divided into three sections. Section I, *Foundation*, provides a history of *Shiatsu* along with that of macrobiotics. Section II explains how to give a complete *Shiatsu*-acupressure treatment—including the loosening phase, designed to increase circulation and relax the body, and the whole body phase, the pressing and massaging of the neck, shoulders, back, abdomen and arms. Section III shows you specific acupressure techniques for over 150 common ailments.

Big Size • Pages: 264
Price: Rs. 150/- • Postage: Rs. 15/-